Hepatitis B

Edited by Luis Rodrigo

Published in London, United Kingdom

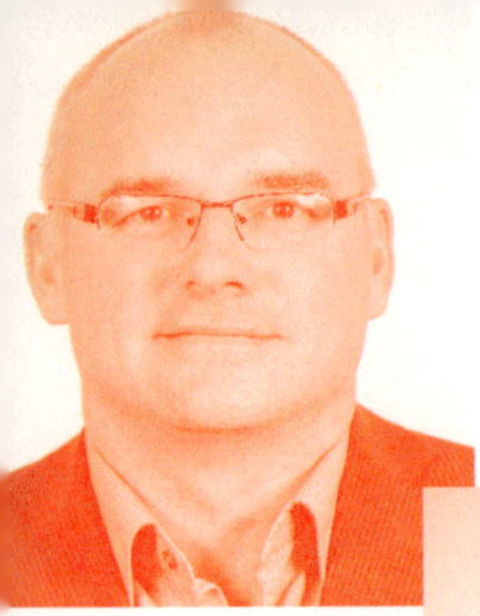
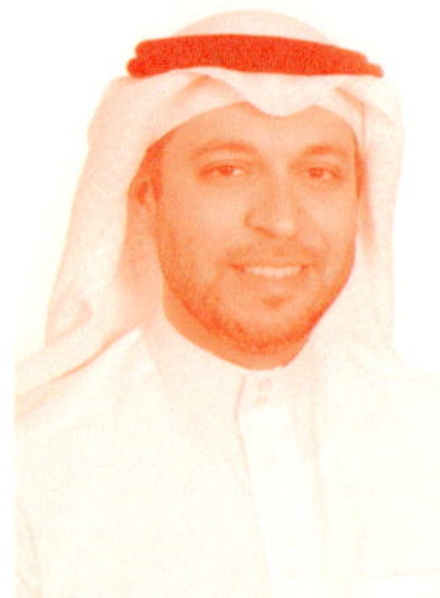
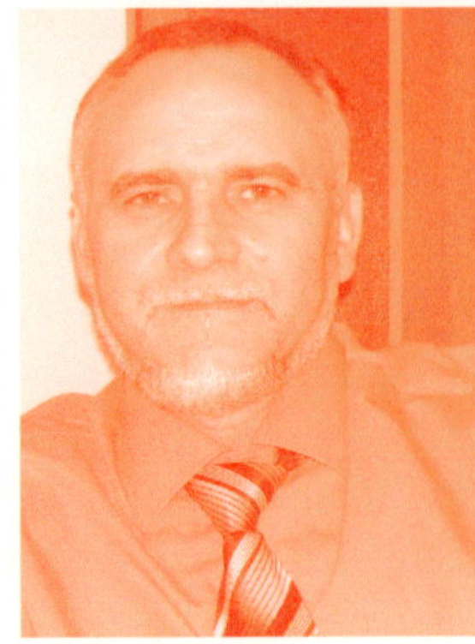
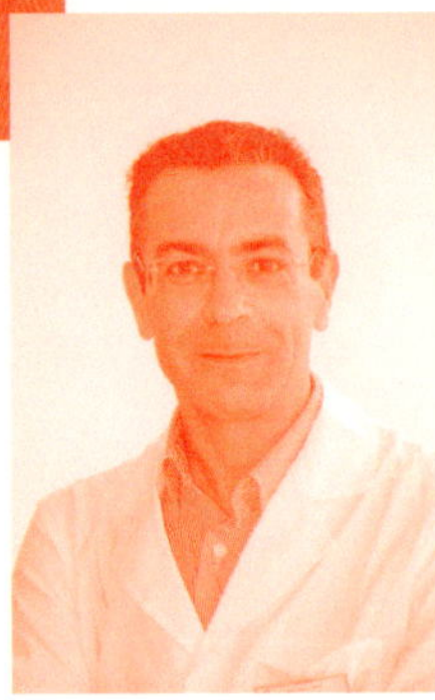
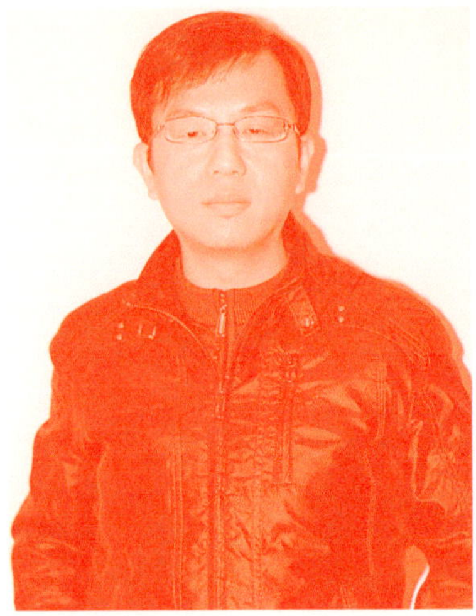
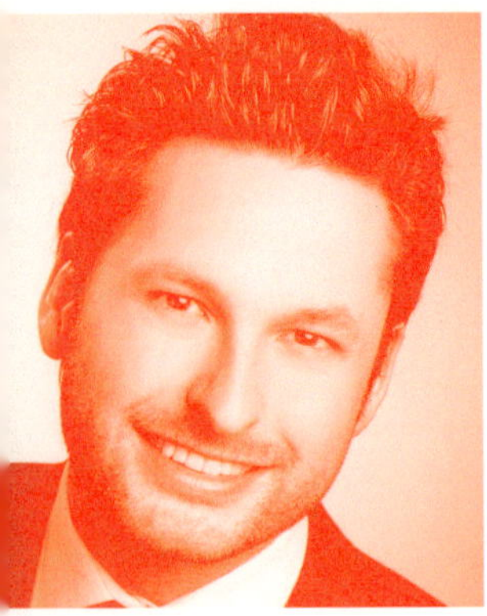
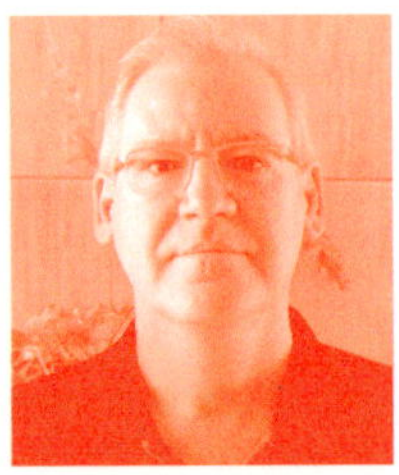

IntechOpen

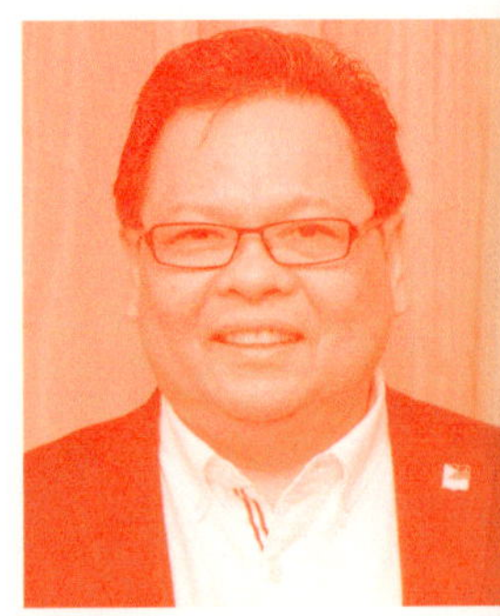
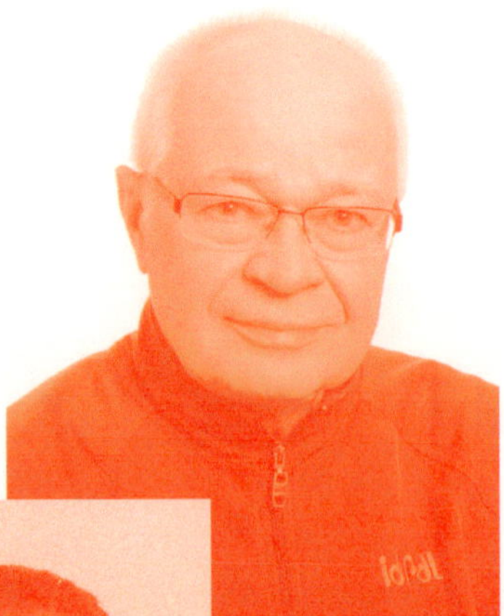
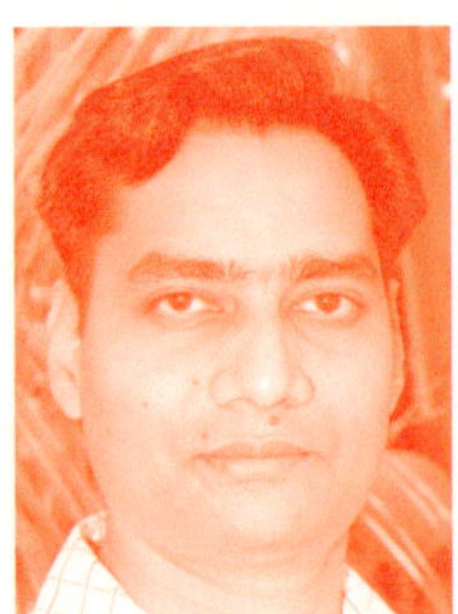
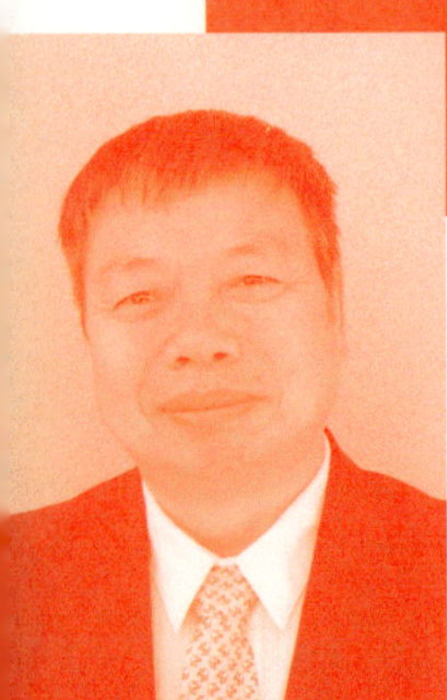
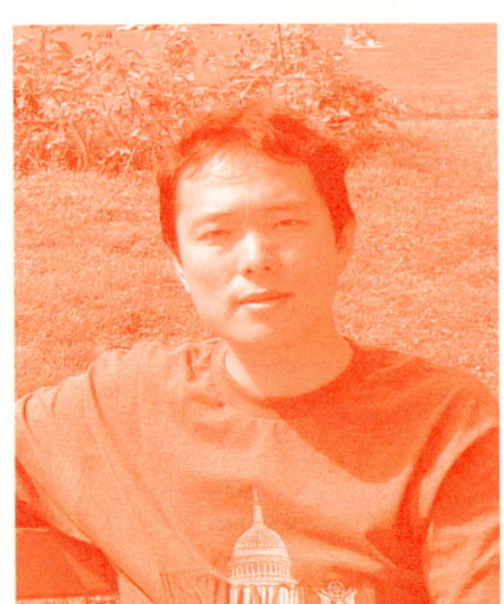
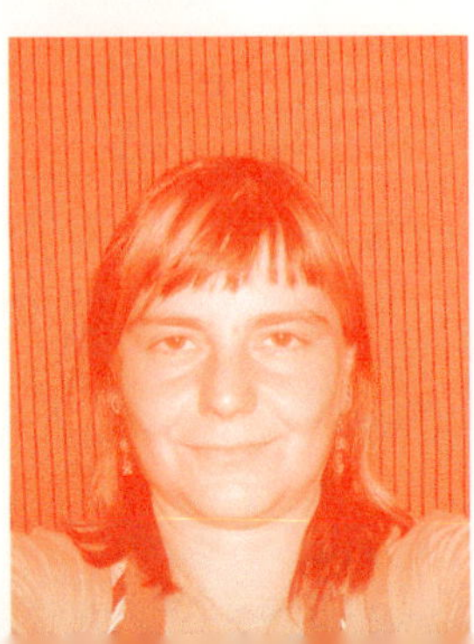

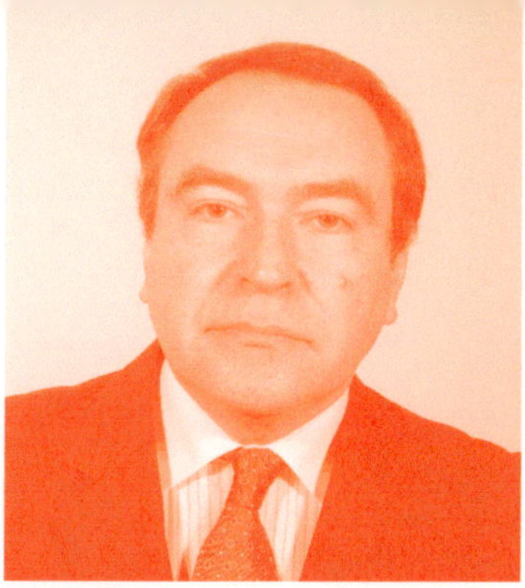
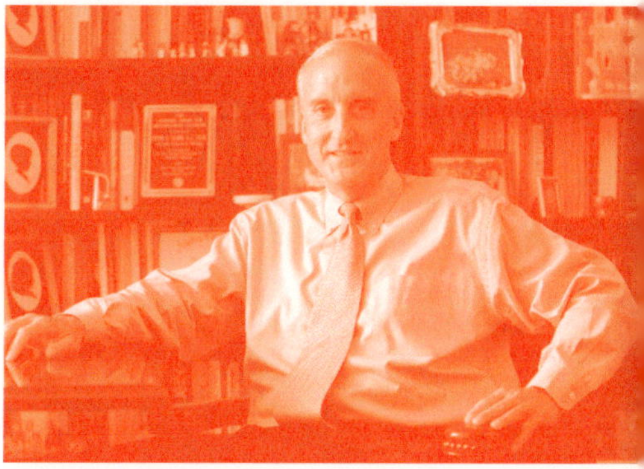
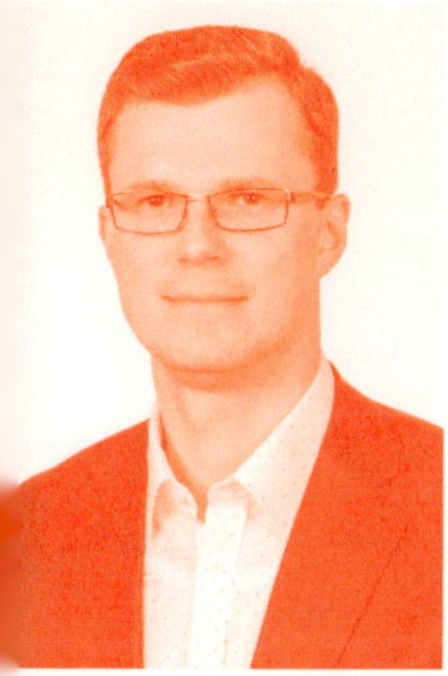
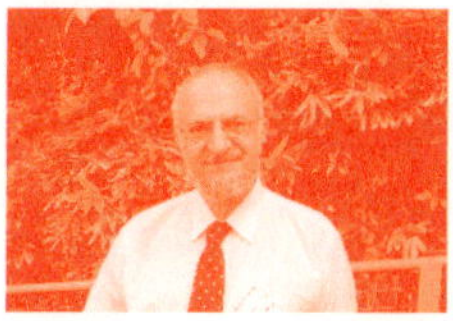
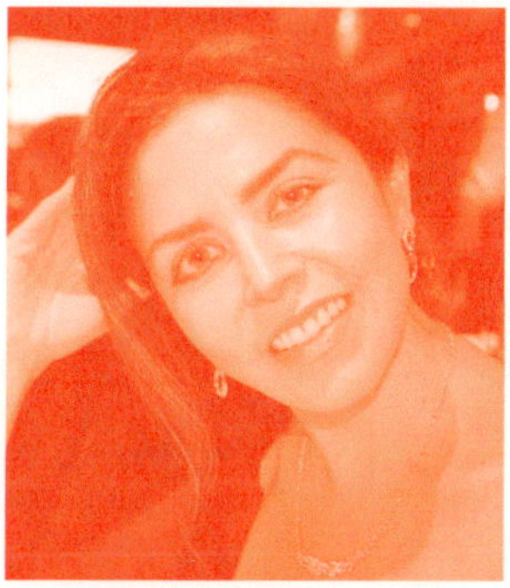

Supporting open minds since 2005

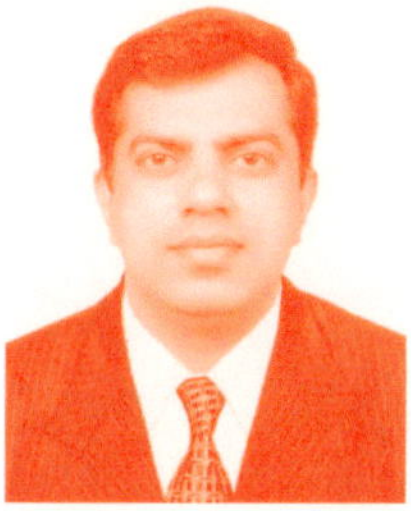
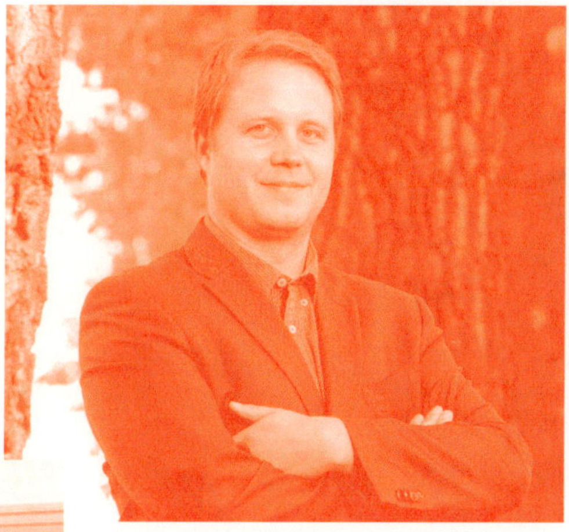
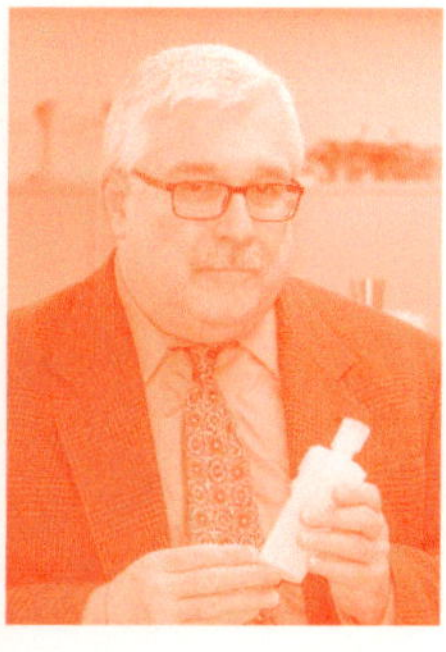
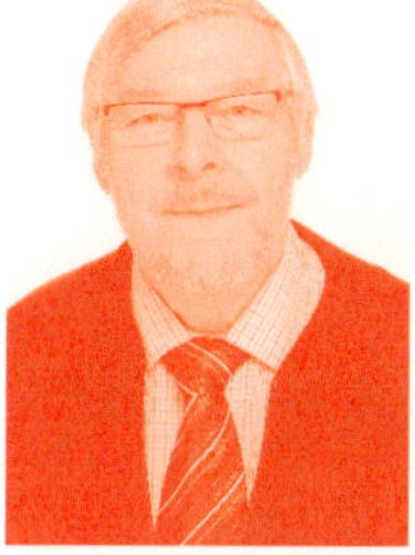
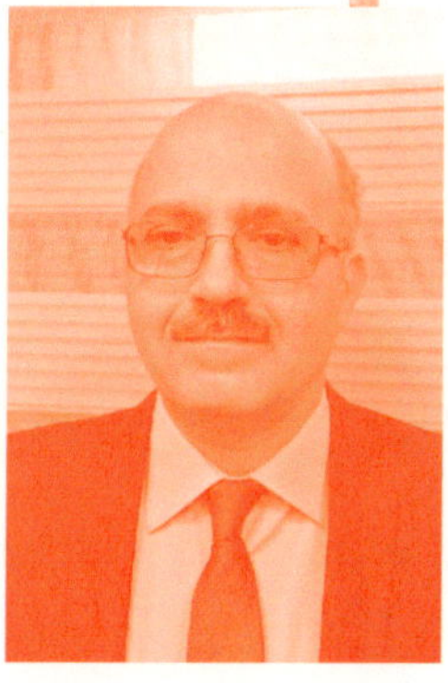
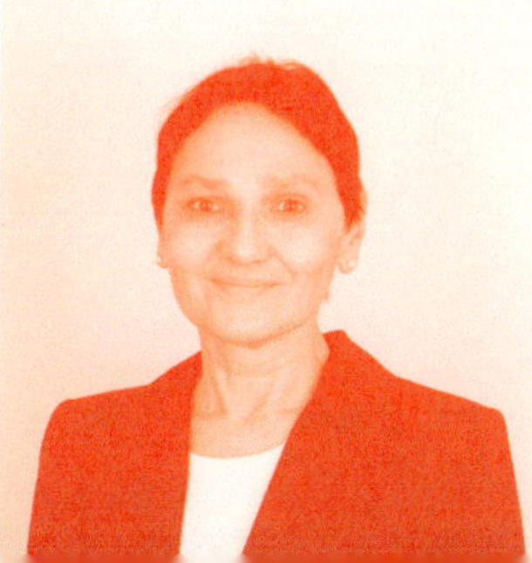
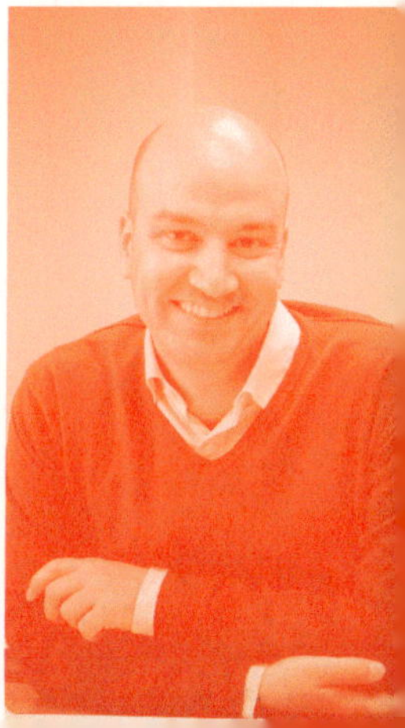

Hepatitis B
http://dx.doi.org/10.5772/intechopen.95726
Edited by Luis Rodrigo

Contributors
Sumit Vallabhdas Bharadva, Avani Shah, Parizad Patel, Kanchan Mishra, Cibangu Katamba, Onoya Onaluwa Philippe, Habtamu Biazin Biazin, Seifegebriel Teshome, Ali Adel Dawood, Yan Yan, Chantsalmaa Davgadorj

First published in London, United Kingdom, 2022 by IntechOpen
IntechOpen is the global imprint of INTECHOPEN LIMITED, registered in England and Wales, registration number: 11086078, 5 Princes Gate Court, London, SW7 2QJ, United Kingdom
Printed in Croatia

British Library Cataloguing-in-Publication Data
A catalogue record for this book is available from the British Library

Additional hard and PDF copies can be obtained from orders@intechopen.com

Hepatitis B
Edited by Luis Rodrigo
p. cm.
Print ISBN 978-1-80355-006-0
Online ISBN 978-1-80355-007-7
eBook (PDF) ISBN 978-1-80355-008-4

For EU product safety concerns:
IN TECH d.o.o., Prolaz Marije Krucifikse Kozulić 3, 51000 Rijeka, Croatia, info@intechopen.com or visit our website at intechopen.com.

Meet the editor

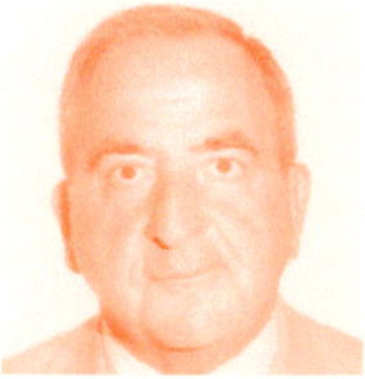

Dr. Luis Rodrigo, MD, is a Professor Emeritus of Medicine, at the University of Oviedo, Spain. He has been Chief of Gastroenterology Service at HUCA Hospital, Oviedo, for more than forty years. He obtained a Ph.D. in 1975 and has developed a long teaching and research career. Dr. Rodrigo has published 716 scientific papers, 435 written in English and the rest in Spanish. He has participated as the main investigator in forty-five clinical trials and has directed forty doctoral theses. He has contributed actively to the formation of around 100 specialists in gastroenterology working in his hospital and other hospitals in Spain and abroad. He has written around thirty-five book chapters and edited twenty-six books in his specialty and related diseases.

Contents

Preface

Hepatitis is inflammation of the liver that can result from a variety of causes such as heavy alcohol use, autoimmune disease, drugs, or toxins. However, the most frequent cause of hepatitis is a viral infection, known as viral hepatitis.

Acute hepatitis is self-resolving in most cases but can cause fulminant liver failure depending on the etiology. In contrast, chronic hepatitis can cause liver damage that includes liver fibrosis, cirrhosis, hepatocellular carcinoma (HCC), and features of portal hypertension leading to significant morbidity and mortality.

Worldwide, hepatitis B and hepatitis C viruses (HBV and HCV) are the most relevant causative viral agents of chronic hepatitis (inflammation of the liver). At present, more than 250 million people suffer from a chronic HBV infection globally, resulting in 0.8 million deaths per year.

Chronic HCV infection accounts for about 70 million cases worldwide, leading to a death toll of about 1 million per year. An approved vaccine is only available against an HBV infection.

Both HBV and HCV infections result in a highly increased risk of developing liver fibrosis, cirrhosis, and HCC. This book describes the mechanisms of HBV and associated pathogenesis.

The book's focus is on the interplay between chronic infection with intracellular signaling transduction, metabolic pathways with an emphasis on lipid metabolism, the establishment of liver fibrosis and cirrhosis during chronic infection, and the mechanisms of the onset of virally induced HCC.

Despite there being great advances in the characterization of viral life cycles and the development of robust antiviral strategies, significant hurdles persist in gaining a better understanding of the mechanisms that drive virus-associated pathogenesis as well as increasing insights regarding different viral genotypes having impacts on alternate pathogeneses.

The first experimental vaccinations against HBV were performed in 1970, even before the nature of the administered "Australia antigen" was known. Soon, it was realized that this antigen was the envelope protein (HBV surface antigen, HBsAg), and it was purified from HBV-containing human plasma. Later, it was produced in genetically engineered yeast cells.

The excellent efficacy of the HBsAg vaccine was confirmed in numerous studies, particularly in newborns from HBV-infected mothers who almost always become chronic HBV carriers without vaccination. The vaccine is also highly effective in older children and adults and has been applied worldwide since 1984, leading to about a tenfold decrease in HBV infections in the vaccinated.

Chronic HBV infection is one of the most common factors associated with HCC, which is the sixth most prevalent cancer among all cancers worldwide. However, the pathogenesis of HBV-mediated hepatocarcinogenesis is unclear. Evidence currently available suggests that the HBV core protein (HBc) plays a potential role in the development of HCC, such as the HBV X protein.

The core protein, which is the structural component of the viral nucleocapsid, contributes to almost every stage of the HBV life cycle and occupies diverse roles in HBV replication and pathogenesis.

Recent studies have shown that HBc was able to disrupt various pathways involved in liver carcinogenesis, including the signaling pathways implicated in migration and proliferation of hepatoma cells, apoptosis pathways, and cell metabolic pathways inducing the development of HCC, and the immune system, through the expression and production of proinflammatory cytokines.

The future of a cure for HBV lies in triple combination therapies with concerted action on replication inhibition, antigen reduction, and immune stimulation. Many obstacles remain, such as overcoming translational failures, choosing the right endpoint using the right biomarkers, and leveraging current treatments in combination regimens to enhance response rates.

In this book, the authors present current therapies for CHB, HBV biomarkers used to evaluate treatment response, and the development of direct-acting antivirals (DAAs) and immune-targeting drugs and discuss the limitations and unanswered questions on the journey to an HBV cure.

Luis Rodrigo MD
Professor,
Emeritus Professor of Medicine,
University of Oviedo,
Oviedo, Spain

Section 1

Epidemiology, Genotypes and Subtypes

Chapter 1

Epidemiology of Hepatitis B Virus

Cibangu Katamba and Onoya Onaluwa Philippe

Abstract

Hepatitis B virus (HBV) is a double-stranded DNA hepadnavirus. It is an important cause of acute 5and chronic hepatitis and hepatocellular carcinoma. Worldwide about 2 billion people show serological evidence of exposure and about 400 million have active infection. High prevalence areas include sub-Saharan Africa, China, and southeast Asia. HBV was known at onset as the etiology of what is called "serum hepatitis", this is the most common form of viral hepatitis transmitted parenterally. It is also a cause of both acute and chronic hepatitis of great significance. Hepatitis B virus has an incubation period that varies between 1 and 6 months. The clinical features of acute infection resemble those of the other viral hepatitides. Death from fulminant hepatitis occurs in about 1%. Following acute infection, there is either complete recovery (with long-term immunity) or persistent infection. The latter occurs in 5–10% infected adults, 30% infected children and 90% infants infected at birth; it is more common in the immunocompromised.

Keywords: hepatitis B, viral hepatitis, epidemiology, incidence, prevalence, distribution

1. Introduction

Hepatitis B Virus (HBV) is a double-stranded DNA hepadnavirus. It is an important cause of acute and chronic hepatitis and hepatocellular carcinoma. Worldwide about 2 billion people show serological evidence of exposure and about 400 million have active infection. High prevalence areas include sub-Saharan Africa, China, and Southeast Asia [1, 2].

HBV has remained a public health issue of global concern in the presence of multiple efforts to eradicate this viral disease through individualized and mass screening, education, and immunization programs [3]. The current estimates have shown that about 400 million individuals throughout the world have chronic HBV infection [1, 3]. Those infected with HBV have 15–40% risk of developing complications such as cirrhosis, hepatic failure, or hepatocellular carcinoma (HCC); and 15–25% of them have the risk of death from related HBV liver disease. About 60–80% of people are diagnosed with HCC and 500,000–1.2 million people die every year due to chronic HBV infection. It is established that HBV infection is the 10th leading cause of death globally.

HBV was known at onset as the etiology of what is called "serum hepatitis", this is the most common form of viral hepatitis transmitted parenterally. It is also a cause of both acute and chronic hepatitis of great significance [4]. Hepatitis B virus has an incubation period that varies between 1 and 6 months. The clinical features of acute infection resemble those of the other viral hepatitides. Death from fulminant hepatitis occurs in about 1%. Following acute infection, there is either complete recovery (with long-term immunity) or persistent infection. The latter occurs in 5–10% infected adults, 30% infected children and 90% infants infected at birth; it is more common in the immunocompromised.

The prevalence of HBV infection varies widely [1–7], with rates ranging from 0.1–20% in different parts of the world. There is high prevalence of hepatitis B surface antigen (HBsAg) positivity rates above 8% in areas of high viral infection endemic prevalence such as the Far East, Sub-Sahara in Africa, the Amazon basin, and some parts of the Middle East. In these settings, there is presence of serologic evidence of prior hepatitis B virus infection anti-hepatitis B core antigen in most cases: positive anti-HBc or anti-HBs. Regions such as India, Japan, Middle East, Eastern & Southern Europe, parts of central Asia and south America are areas with intermediate chronic HBV infection prevalence (2–7% positive HBsAg). The regions with low chronic HBV infection prevalence (below 2percent positive HBsAg) include the USA, Australia, Southern South America, and Northern Europe. Throughout the world 45% of the global population live in high prevalence areas generally. People immigrating from high to low endemic regions have shown patterns that have a greater impact on the epidemiology of HBV; e.g., Migration of individuals from countries in South East Asia resulted in increased prevalence of chronic hepatitis B in the USA.

2. Modes of transmission of hepatitis B virus

We have two major modes of transmission of hepatitis B virus in the world [1–3]: perinatal and horizontal transmissions. The perinatal transmission occurs during child delivery from infected mothers to their babies, this mode of spread accounts for the majority of transmissions in the world. The second mode is horizontal transmission, that can occur through open wounds (cuts and scratches), blood transfusion, poor infection prevention practices to curve blood-borne infections in health facilities, sexual transmission and risky health behaviors such as piercing of the body, unsafe drugs injection, body tattoos and scarification using unsterilized instruments & other equipment. Developing chronic hepatitis B virus infection depends on the mode of spread of the virus, as the risk decreases with age at infection for susceptible individuals. About 90% of infections acquired during perinatal period will become chronical. Up to 20–60% of under 5 infections (1 to below 5 years of age) and 5–10% of adults and older children will develop chronic HBV infection.

Hepatitis B virus can be found in body fluids such as blood, saliva, vaginal fluids and menses, semen; and in less amount in breast milk, perspiration, urine, tears of infected people. HBV is easily spread through contact with body secretions, the virus resists to breakdown and can live long outside the human body. Heterosexual & other sexual activities and unsafe use of drugs by people who inject drugs account for most transmissions of the virus in regions with low prevalence.

Vertical or perinatal transmission of HBV is commonly observed in countries in the Far East Asian and Oceania regions. Mothers with high viral load have higher chances of transmitting the virus to their new born. Infection during child birth occurs in 5–20% of babies born to HBsAg positive, HBeAg-negative women. While most perinatal infections occur in babies born to chronically infected mothers, those with acute HBV infection in the 3rd trimester are also very likely to transmit the virus. Only less than 2% of perinatal transmissions occur in-utero.

The horizontal transmission during early childhood is significant in some regions in particular Sub-Saharan Africa, Alaska, and the Mediterranean, where perinatal transmission is less common as compared to Asia. There is lower prevalence of positive HBeAg correlates in mothers with less efficient spread during child birth. Nonetheless, by the time the child is 10 years old, about 90% of children in rural Sub-Saharan regions of Africa will show evidence of past exposure to the virus. In the same population, HBeAg wean off in early in contrast to Asians, and most of them are HBeAg-negative by the reproductive age.

There is a possibility that these observations in epidemiologic variations are secondary to genotypic differences in hepatitis B virus. The accurate mode of spread in early childhood is not known, it is however thought that it occurs through blood and body secretions (not apparent) from family members or peers/playmates that inoculate the virus into cuts (scratches or abrasions) to the skin or other mucosal lesions.

The laboratory tests specific for HBV have revealed the fact that transmission through blood and blood products, and parenteral transmissions seem to be especially blood related. It is however important to note that infectivity does not solely appear by blood-to-blood contact. It has been observed that certain experimentations render the viral transmission by mouth is ineffective. The infection may be endemic in semi-closed and closed settings and mentally handicapped facilities. It is more common in urban settings among adults and those living in deprived socio-economic states. Marked differences can be observed for the infection prevalence and the carrier states in various geographical areas and between people with different ethnic and socio-economic statuses.

Enough evidence exists to show the transmission of HBV by intimate and sexual contacts. People who are sexually promiscuous, especially those active homosexual males who change partners regularly, have very high chances of acquiring hepatitis B virus infection. The surface antigen for HBV has been detected in blood and various body secretions like semen, menses and vaginal fluids, saliva, breast milk (including colostrum) and serous fluids. These body fluids have been implicated in the transmission of the virus. Therefore, hepatitis through contact is of major importance. The virus may be accidentally transmitted from inoculation of small amount of blood or fluids contaminated with blood during medical or surgical interventions, vaccination with inadequately sterilized equipment such as needles and syringes, drug-injections, tattooing, piercing of ear and nose, acupuncture, razors, shared toothbrushes, towels and other linens contaminated with blood. Other factors related to transmission in specific climates in the tropics and warn-countries are important to note; including ritual circumcision, blood-letting, repeated bites by bloodsucking arthropod vectors, traditional tattooing and scarification. However, findings on the role which biting insects play in the transmission of HBV are conflicting. HBsAg has been detected in multiple species of mosquito and bedbugs either trapped in the wild or fed experimentally on infected blood in laboratories. No convincing outcome for replication of hepatitis B virus in insect has been shown. Also, there is no evidence in epidemiology for mechanical transmission of HBV by insects.

HBsAg has been reported present in feces, urine and bile, often as a result of blood contamination. HBV is not known to be transmitted through fecal-oral mode and urine. Urine is not infectious unless it is blood contaminated. There is no evidence to show airborne transmission of the infection. Clustering of HBV can be seen in family settings but this is not associated with genetic factors and does not imply venereal or maternal transmission. The mechanisms of HBV intrafamilial transmission is yet to be established.

3. Donation of tissues and blood

As a standard of care, blood donors are now universally screened for hepatitis B with HBsAg test [1]. This had markedly reduced the risk of infection transmission through transfusion. Countries around the world with negligible prevalence have also added anti-HBc tests to detect chronic carriers with low viral load who may not be detected with HBsAg test. These two tests decrease HBV infection rates to about 2.5–15.3 per million units of blood in settings with low prevalence rates. Developed countries like Canada, USA, Australia, Japan, etc. perform other more sensitive tests/nucleic acid tests additionally. However, the benefits in terms of incremental yield and other clinical advantages of nucleic acid tests over rapid tests (serologic) in these regions with low HBV prevalence, and the need for additional serologic tests, has not been established. Since about 90% of adults individuals have serologic evidence of ongoing or past HBV infection, anti-HBc is not to be used as a screening test in settings with high burden of hepatitis B. Therefore, in these settings, HBsAg is the only screening test being used. Nevertheless, in these settings, occult hepatitis B is seen in 3–30% of people with positive HBc and negative HBsAg. We now know that HBsAg-negative, positive hepatitis B DNA blood carries about 10% risk of transmission. In Taiwan, the risk of transmission of Hepatitis B infection through transfusion was approximated recently to be 100 per million units, with donor screening strategy using HBsAg test alone. This means that it is 7–40 times higher than in settings with low prevalence. The nucleic acid tests had a yield estimated to be at least 20 times higher in settings with high prevalence as compared to those with low prevalence, where it is currently in use. This has rendered it more cost saving per infection averted in these settings. Anti-HBc screening test is strategy is more cost-effective compared to nucleic acid tests in areas with lo prevalence despite the potential role of nucleic acid testing in these areas. The sensitivity and specificity of nucleic acid tests vary in most high prevalence settings. There is need to develop newer HBsAg assays with improved sensitivity to address this issue.

The other potential spread of occult or subclinical hepatitis B virus is from tissues and organs donation. Undetected viral load at time of tissue donation may be more frequent among tissue donors than blood donors according to estimates. To prevent infection following tissue or organ transplant, the easiest way is to exclude HBc-positive donors. This approach may not be practical in settings with high prevalence where most people have prior exposure to the virus. Consequently, the nucleic acid test is good additional measure to screening strategies for tissue donors to reduce the chances of transmission. The challenge, however, remains to reduce the turnaround time for results of nucleic acid test performed in clinical transplant facilities.

4. Mother to child transmission

HBV can be transmitted to infants born from carrier mothers during child labour and delivery. This is the single most important factor that determines the prevalence of HBV infection in some settings, especially the Southern parts of Eastern Asia and China. The chances of acquiring HBV infection in infant may approximate 90% and seem to be associated with ethnic groups. Pediatric infections are particularly important because a big number of these infants will be carriers. Hepatitis B infectivity is directly associated with the presence of high titres of HBsAg and/or HBeAg in the mother's blood stream. About95% of new born babies are infected around delivery time when HBeAg is present in their mother's circulation. The prevalence of HBeAg among mothers who carry the virus as well as mother to child' infectivity varies significantly in various settings and ethnic groups.

In South-East Asia, about 30–50% of HBsAg carrier mothers also carry HBeAg in their circulation. Perinatal transmissions are estimated to account for about 50% of the carriers in this population. These infections are frequent in babies born from mother of West Asian and Afro-Caribbean decent. In the contrary, Caucasian women present fewer perinatal transmissions and carrier states. Mother to child transmission of infection and the carrier state patterns are different in regions such as Africa, where HBeAg is less common in carriers and the infection to their babies is frequently seen during the first 5 years of life resulting in horizontal transmission. The transmission of hepatitis B infection to infants born from non-carrier women by contact with other playmates who are infected from their carrier mothers is another mode of spread of the virus.

The considerable risk of hepatitis B infection during perinatal period from mothers with acute HBV infection is possible, especially during the 3rd trimester or within 2 months post-delivery. Transmission in-utero is not common, since HBV does not cross the intact placenta and the limited number of intrauterine infections are probably due to maternal blood leakage into the fetal blood stream associated with a tear in the placenta.

The exact mechanism of infection during perinatal period is not known but it is probable that this happens during delivery or shortly after birth due to maternal blood leakage into the fetal blood stream or the ingestion/inadvertent inoculation of maternal blood into the baby's circulation. The majority of infants infected during labour and delivery become chronic carriers.

HBeAg is a serologic marker for hepatitis B DNA viral load. Infections during perinatal period occur almost always in mothers who are positive for hepatitis B but can also occur in women who have very high viral load, hepatitis B virus DNA greater than 200,000 IU/ml in their blood. If the child is not immunized, his/her risk of acquiring hepatitis B virus during delivery is almost 100% when the mother has a positive HBeAg. The famous Taiwan study by Palmer Beasley as reported by Zuckerman [1] in the 1970s when there was no vaccine available showed that 85% of positive HBeAg mothers had their babies developing chronic infection vs only 32% of the negative ones. There is an approximated 90% risk of infants who acquired infection during perinatal period becoming chronically infected.

To reduce mother to child transmission of hepatitis B virus, incorporating the birth immunization dose into the HBV immunization schedule is the most effective strategy. This dose, if followed by two more doses, can significantly reduce the prevalence of chronic infection in babies born from positive HBeAg mothers by about 90%, and by about 100% from negative HBeAg mothers. The birth dose is particularly important in in settings were an important proportion of mothers with positive HBsAg and positive HBeAg at the same time. Such settings include the Pacific Islands, South East-Asia, and China. In these regions, if the birth dose is missed, HBV vaccine' effectiveness could reduce to about 50–75%. In other areas of the world such as Sub-Sahara in Africa, and Russia where less than 25% of pregnant mothers with a positive HBsAg have also positive HBeAg, the consequences of missing the birth dose are still significant but not as severe. The expended immunization program should include a dose of hepatitis B immunoglobulin at birth to babies born to mothers with positive HBsAg. This has the potential to reduce further the chances of transmission to below 5%. A randomized controlled trial by Beasley et al. demonstrated that the birth dose of hepatitis B immunoglobulin administered to babies born to mothers with both positive HBsAg and HBeAg lead to only 6% of these babies seroconverting to positive HBsAg as compared to 88% of babies in the placebo arm.

5. Horizontal spread

The horizontal spread of hepatitis B virus is very likely to lead to chronic state if it occurs in young children [1, 3, 6]. This was demonstrated in several studies conducted before the HBV vaccine was made available. Research conducted in Senegal revealed that half the children who had horizontal transmission of HBV before they were 2 years old developed chronic infection. In another research on 1280 people who had hepatitis B virus negative sero-markers in rural Alaskan conducted in the 1970s revealed that 29% of children below 5 years old, out of 189 individuals who acquired the infection over a four-year period, had chronic hepatitis B against 16% of children between 5 and 10 years old, and only 8% for adults above 30 years old. The birth dose of hepatitis B vaccine together with the subsequent doses can reduce the acquisition of infection in the early months of life as well as prevent perinatal transmission in settings where the risk of chronicity through horizontal transmission of the infection is great.

Horizontal transmission, if it occurs in young children and some adults, this is because of high likelihood of infectious hepatitis B virus found on surfaces. The research conducted in Alaska many years ago, before the availability of viral DNA testing, the hepatitis B surface antigen was found in the environment on samples from table tops from school lunch room, toys, feeding bottles, and walls in houses where positive HBsAg individuals lived. Hepatitis B viral replication was possible at room temperature after at least 7 days. There is possibility that the virus can be spread through broken skin and mucosa from people with chronic infection on to surfaces, infecting thereby other people with open lesions. The horizontal transmission can also happen through non-sterile objects and procedures such as injections from healthcare providers or drug-injection, tattooing, scarification, sexual route, dialysis, emergency procedures, etc.

Young adults in the USA have increased horizontal transmission of HBV through unsafe drug-injection use in some places. There was 114% increase in the acute hepatitis B infection between 2006 and 2013 in West Virginia, Kentucky, and Tennessee. This increase was seen mostly in white populations between 30 and 39 years old who had a drug-injection history. In health care facilities, the outbreaks of hepatitis B can also increase the horizontal spread of the virus. The prevention of horizontal spread entails the combination of several measure such as education, good infection prevention and control practices, and immunization of household contacts to hepatitis B infected individuals and other people at high risk of HBV infection.

5.1 Vaccination

Hepatitis B vaccine is now available for over decades now. It is highly effective infection prevention measure among people at high risk of developing the disease [8]. The USA implemented universal immunization in 1991 and saw the incidence of acute infection decrease by 89% in adolescents and young children. With this exercise, the disparities in prevalence of chronic hepatitis B infection between races have reduced. Hepatitis B virus is endemic in Alaska, but following immunization, the incidence of new infections has markedly decreased. With this achievement, the incidence of hepatic cirrhosis and hepatocellular carcinoma is expected to reduce as well in the next few decades. Taiwan is one of the nations that adopted universal vaccination earlier. Its prevalence of positive surface antigen than was between 15–20% has reduced to 7% among adolescents and young children.

6. Chronic carriers

The concept "carrier state" is defined as persistence of HBsAg in blood circulation for more than 6 months, based on longitudinal researches. This state maybe associated hepatic changes comprising minor damage in the nuclei of liver cells to persistent liver inflammation, chronic active hepatitis, liver cirrhosis, and hepatocellular carcinoma. The integration of the HBV DNA may occur at several places or at unique site of the host genome in carriers of HBV with or without histological evidence of hepatic disease. The majority of carriers have HBsAg in their circulation with or without other markers of the viral infection (HBeAg, HBV DNA, DNA polymerase). The continued expression of HBsAg is suggestive of integrated viral DNA resultant. Some HBV carriers may have HBV DNA in their liver but with no surface antigen expression, this is called "latent viral infection".

There are a number of risk factors that have been established in accordance to the "carrier state". The carrier state is most common in male gender, it is more likely to follow infections acquired in childhood than those acquired in adulthood, it occurs most often in individuals with natural or acquired immune deficiencies. The carrier state develops in only about 5–10% of infections acquired in adult life.

Carriers' prevalence among adults who appear healthy, especially the blood donors vary by region. The global population can be grouped in to three regions by prevalence of hepatitis B virus infection:

a. Hyperendemic regions: here, the infection includes almost always several countries of South-East Asia, China, the Western Pacific, and the sub-Saharan region of Africa. In these settings, infection in early life is very common. The proportions of carriers in these regions range from above 5–20%.

b. Intermediate endemic regions: here, the prevalence of hepatitis B infection range from 20–50% generally (by serologic markers like HBsAg, anti-HBs and anti-HBc), and that of carriers from 1–5% overall. It is seen in countries in the Northern region of Africa, the middle East, South America, and parts of Southern and Eastern Europe.

c. Low prevalence regions: here, less than 10% of the general population have evidence of hepatitis B virus infection by serologic markers, and a carrier rate of less than 0.1%. Nevertheless, the prevalence of HBV infection and carriers vary considerably in these settings within ethnic groups. These regions include northern Europe, the USA, Canada, most Western Europe, New Zealand, and Australia.

With the advent of HIV/AIDS, the hepatitis B virus coinfection with HIV has become a major concern of late because of synergic negative effects of both viruses. HIV coinfection increase the chances of hepatic disease progression related to hepatitis B virus while hepatitis B coinfection augment antiretroviral therapy related liver toxicity.

7. Distribution of hepatitis B by age

It has been recognized two different patterns of hepatitis B infection by age distribution [1, 8, 9]. Individuals with high burden of HBV, infection is often acquired early during childhood. The highest infection and carrier rates are usually seen among children and young adults while the lowest is prevalent among older individuals. The HBeAg has been found more frequently in young carriers than in their adult counterparts. In contrast, HBe antibody is more common in older individuals. These results are in keeping with the possibility of young carriers being most infective.

In settings where this viral infection is not commonly observed, the highest prevalence of HBsAg occurs in populations between the age of 20 and 40 years old. The highest rates of hepatitis B infections are seen in populations at increased risk of contact with blood or blood products, e.g., health care workers, certain groups of patients, IV drug users, and male promiscuous homosexuals.

There is need to understand that the prevalence of hepatitis B infection, the age distribution of this infection, the carrier state. This change is drastic in some regions with the implementation of routine program of expanded hepatitis B vaccination.

8. Hepatitis B genotypes

There are six HBV genotypes grouped A-F based on phylogenetic analysis of complete viral genome classification [10, 11]. The most disseminated genotypes throughout the world are A and D. In contrast, B and C genotypes are restricted to East Asia, and E genotype to sub-Saharan Africa. The genotype F on the other hand is more diverse from other genotype classes and is seen in aboriginal Americans. All the genotype classes have a common immunodominant area on the surface antigen that is called "a determinant". This determinant span amino acids 124–147 and is hydrophilic. It is taught to be a form of two major and one minor loops with cysteine disulphide bonds. The "a" determinant target primarily the neutralizing antibodies induced by vaccination. The available hepatitis B vaccines have common major immunization response to "a" epitope with subsequent protection against all subtypes of HBV.

9. Burden of HBV in developing countries

HBV has an intermediate to high endemicity levels in developing countries [12–16]. Recently, the incidence of acute infection has decreased in several countries. The prevalence of chronic carriers of HBsAg has also decreased, this is as a result of the introduction of universal immunization coverage for hepatitis B virus in the 1990s. A few other countries are still not able to implement these interventions, especially in their rural and highly endemic regions. There is lack of sufficient information on the epidemiology of hepatitis B virus in many Eastern Europe and Latin-America countries.

9.1 Epidemiology

9.1.1 Africa

The entire Africa is known to be highly endemic continent for hepatitis B virus. The infection occurs with more than 8% hyperendemicity for chronic carriers of surface antigen in the general population in countries of Sub-Sahara like Nigeria, Cameroon, Burkina Faso, Gabon, and Namibia. Some other countries such as Zambia, Kenya, Senegal, Ivory Coast, Liberia, and Sierra Leone experience intermediate endemicity (2–8%). The following countries are considered to have low HBV endemicity (below 2%) in Africa: Morocco, Algeria, and Egypt.

Children in Africa are at high risk of acquiring hepatitis B infection. The hepatitis B markers seroconversion rates vary from 10.2–60.5% annually in Somalian children between 1 and 10 years old. The highest rates are seen in children with a low socio-economic situation. In South Africa, the highest rate of hepatitis B infection in Children (5–6 years old) was 15.7%. The infection is often acquired by these children through parenteral horizontal transmission route from siblings and parents. Unsafe sharing of toiletries and sharpening, cutting, scraping or scratching instruments in the daily activities accounts for such a high horizontal transmission. In addition, cultural practices like scarification and tattooing and sexual promiscuity greatly increase the chance of hepatitis B infection. Hepatitis B transmission by transfusion of blood and blood products still occurs and is taught to have an epidemiological impact in some regions in Sub-Saharan countries.

9.1.2 Asia

The Arabian region or South-Western Asia accounts for 10% of territories in Asia. The Arabian Peninsula (Saudi Arabia, Bahrain, the Unites Arab Emirates, Oman, and Yemen included) together with Kuwait have a positive e antigen prevalence from 1.5 to above 8%. The HBsAg-positive prevalence in the Gaza Strip is 3.5% in the general population and 3.8% in blood donors.

Arab countries have implemented the WHO-recommended Expanded Program on Immunization, and hepatitis B virus immunization programs started in these countries have now covered a large proportion of their population. This has successfully reduced the hepatitis B virus endemicity.

Saudi Arabia is the first Arab country to adopt an HBV immunization program. It has seen a steady decline in positive surface antigen prevalence observed in children aged between 1 and 12 years, from 7% in 1989 to 0.31% in 1997 and zero% in 2008.

Cambodia is one of the western Pacific countries with the hepatitis B Virus prevalence at 4.6% in the adult population and 6% in blood donors. In this country, high anti-HBc rates have been reported (58.6% and 72.4%) in different studies, suggesting a principal role played in the past by horizontal transmission in childhood and adulthood.

China also started the universal HBV immunization program of newborn babies in 1992. In this country, the prevalence of surface antigen carriers decreased from 9.8% in 1992 to 7.18% in 2006. The immunization coverage rate at the end of 2005 was 20% lower in rural areas than in the urban areas, a difference that has steadily decreased in recent years. China has gone from a high to an intermediate endemicity level in a short period of time despite the suboptimal immunization coverage. The prevalence of anti-HBs was higher in fully immunized children (63.2–74.3%) than in non-immunized subjects (21.1–34.8%) because of the universal hepatitis B immunization campaign.

9.1.3 Eastern Europe

There are very few epidemiological studies conducted on hepatitis B virus infection in Eastern Europe which do not provide conclusive evidence on the spread of hepatitis B at the level of generalization of routine immunization in this large geographic region.

In a recent study from Bulgaria, positive surface antigen prevalence in persons below 20 years old, targeted by hepatitis B immunization, was significantly lower than that found in non-vaccinated persons aged over 20 (1% against 4.8%). The hepatitis B surface antigen-positive seroprevalence in the general population was 3.8% in studies performed in Bulgaria, 5.6% in Romania and from 4.4–13% in different studies in Serbia, with wide variations within single countries that reflect the different socio-economic conditions between rural and urban areas. In these studies, males showed higher rates of hepatitis B surface antigen positivity than females.

9.1.4 Latin America

The epidemiological information on hepatitis B virus is insufficient and in pieces in Latin America. About 7–12 million Latin Americans are carriers of hepatitis B chronic infection according to estimates. The rate of positive surface antigen individuals varies between countries, the highest being recorded in the 20–40 age groups possibly because of horizontal transmission. Recently, progress from intermediate to low endemicity levels have been registered in some tropical countries in Latin America such as Venezuela, Colombia, and Panama. Hepatitis B infection still provides a heavy socioeconomic burden in many developing nations despite universal immunization programs introduced in the 1990s. These programs need to be extended without fail to cover the rural areas in countries where hepatitis B vaccination is demonstrating its efficacy in reducing the transmission of the virus. Countries that are still unable to adopt a universal immunization program for newborn babies need to receive support from international health organizations to implement this.

10. Burden of HBV in the United States

There are approximately 700,000 to greater than 2 million people with chronic HBV infection in the USA. It is difficult to obtain accurate approximations of individuals burdened with chronic HBV infection in the world and in the USA in particular due the asymptomatic nature of the disease in most people infected with the virus [9]. This results in more people not diagnosed, passive surveillance, and underreporting. With the introduction of universal immunization in the USA, there is increased immunity among children and adolescents. Despite this progress, the number of adults infected with chronic hepatitis B has been increasing because of immigration of infected individuals from highly endemic settings. It is estimated that about 70% of hepatitis B infections in the USA are from foreign-born individuals. About 40,000–45,000 subjects from hepatitis B virus endemic settings (with chronic hepatitis B infection prevalence above 2%) immigrate to the USA legally. The total number of immigrants from Eastern Asia and Sub-Saharan Africa living in the USA is estimated above 3.9 million.

The National Health and Examination Survey (NHANES, 2011 & 2012) revealed that about 850,000 Americans are living with Chronic hepatitis B. Non-Hispanic individuals represent approximately 5% of the United States population. The oversampling of this group revealed that about half of all chronic hepatitis B infections (400,000) in the USA are seen among non-Hispanic Asians. The rates of acute hepatitis B infection have remained about 1 per 100,000 population since 2009 in the USA. These have been reported mainly from non-urban as compared to urban areas. The highest rate of acute hepatitis B infection in the USA is reported among African American adult populations. Of late, between 2006 and 2013, there was an increase in incidence of acute hepatitis B infection in Tennessee, West Virginia, and Kentucky, among white populations between the age of 30 and 39 years old who reported common risk factor such as drug-injection use.

DOI: http://dx.doi.org/10.5772/intechopen.101097

Author details

Cibangu Katamba* and Onoya Onaluwa Philippe
Lusaka Provincial Health Office, Lusaka, Zambia

*Address all correspondence to: patrickkatamba@gmail.com

References

[1] Zuckerman AJ, editor. Hepatitis B in the Asian-Pasific Region. Vol. 1-3. London: Royal College of Physicians; 1999

[2] Zanetti AR, Tanzi E, Manzillo G, et al. Hepatitis B variant in Europe. Lancet. 1988;**2**:1132-1133

[3] Nainan O V, Stevens C E, Taylor P E et al. Hepatitis B virus (HBV) antibody resistant mutants among mothers and infants with chronic HBV infection. In: Rizzetto M, Purcell R H, Gerin J L & Verme G (ed) Viral Hepatitis and Liver Disease. Torino: Minerva Medica; 1997 pp. 132-134

[4] Hsu HY, Chang MH, Liaw SH, et al. Changes of hepatitis B surface antigen variants in carrier children before and after universal vaccination in Taiwan. Hepatology. 1999;**30**:1312-1317

[5] Report of a WHO consultation. Global surveillance and control of hepatitis C

[6] Cook GC, Zumla A. Section 6 Viral infections. Chapter 40: Viral hepatitis. In: Zuckerman JN, Zuckerman AJ, editors. Manson's Tropical Diseases. 21st ed. London: Saunders; 2003. pp. 710-713

[7] Eddleston M, Davidson R, Brent A, et al. Oxford Handbook of Tropical Medicine. 3rd ed. Oxford: Oxford; 2007. pp. 294-295

[8] Trépo C, Chan HL, Lok A. Hepatitis B virus infection. Lancet. 2014;**384**(9959):2053-2063. DOI: 10.1016/S0140-6736(14)60220-8. Epub 2014 Jun 18. Available from: https://pubmed.ncbi.nlm.nih.gov/24954675/

[9] Zampino R, Boemio A, Sagnelli C, Alessio L, Adinolfi LE, Sagnelli E, et al. Hepatitis B virus burden in developing countries. World Journal of Gastroenterology. 2015;**21**(42): 11941-11953. DOI: 10.3748/wjg.v21.i42.11941. Available from: https://pubmed.ncbi.nlm.nih.gov/26576083/

[10] Hedley-Whyte J, Milamed DR. Hepatitis B: Prevalence, hope. Ulster Medical Journal. 2019;**88**(2):118-123. Epub 2019 Apr 27. Available from: https://pubmed.ncbi.nlm.nih.gov/31073252/

[11] Alexander J, Kowdley KV. Epidemiology of hepatitis B--Clinical implications. MedGenMed. 2006;**8**(2):13. Available from: https://pubmed.ncbi.nlm.nih.gov/16926752/

[12] Katamba C, Chungu T, Lusale C. HIV, syphilis and hepatitis B coinfections in Mkushi, Zambia: A cross-sectional study. F1000Research. 2019;**8**:562. DOI: 10.12688/f1000research.17983.2. Available from: https://www.ncbi.nlm.nih.gov/pmc/articles/PMC7417957/

[13] Nelson NP, Easterbrook PJ, BJ MM. Epidemiology of hepatitis B virus infection and impact of vaccination on disease. Clinical Liver Disease. 2016;**20**(4):607-628. DOI: 10.1016/j.cld.2016.06.006. Erratum in: Clinical Liver Disease. 2017;**21**(2):xiii. Available from: https://pubmed.ncbi.nlm.nih.gov/27742003/

[14] Ott JJ, Stevens GA, Groeger J, Wiersma ST. Global epidemiology of hepatitis B virus infection: New estimates of age-specific HBsAg seroprevalence and endemicity. Vaccine. 2012;**30**(12):2212-2219. DOI: 10.1016/j.vaccine.2011.12.116. Epub 2012 Jan 24. Available from: https://pubmed.ncbi.nlm.nih.gov/22273662/

[15] Nguyen MH, Wong G, Gane E, Kao JH, Dusheiko G. Hepatitis B virus: Advances in prevention, diagnosis, and therapy. Clinical Microbiology Reviews. 2020;**33**(2):e00046-e00019.

DOI: 10.1128/CMR.00046-19. Available from: https://pubmed.ncbi.nlm.nih.gov/32102898/

[16] Sunbul M. Hepatitis B virus genotypes: Global distribution and clinical importance. World Journal of Gastroenterology. 2014;**20**(18):5427-5434. DOI: 10.3748/wjg.v20.i18.5427. Available from: https://pubmed.ncbi.nlm.nih.gov/24833873/

Chapter 2

Hepatitis B Virus, Genotypes and Subtypes

Ali Adel Dawood

Abstract

Hepatitis simply means inflammation of liver. This word came from heap: the Latin for liver and "titis" means inflammation. In addition to viruses, many varieties of agents can cause hepatitis such as bacteria, parasites, fungi and chemical agents including drugs, toxins and alcohol. Hepatitis B virus is classified as an Orthohepadna virus (Genera) within the family *Hepadnaviridae*. This family Includes the wood chuck hepatitis virus WHV, the duck hepatitis virus DHBV, and several other avian and mammalian variants. The human HBV has been shown to infect chimpanzees, Barbary macaques and tree shrews. All hepadnaviridae have similar to hepatotropism and life cycles in their hosts. HBV infection is a global health problem which is 50–100 times more infectious than HIV. Approximately 400 million people are carriers of chronic liver disease every year due to consequences of the disease. Not only HBV can infect hepatocytes but also infects in extrahepatic sites including lymph nodes, bone marrow, circulating lymphocytes, spleen and pancreas. Hepatitis B virus can occur as an acute or chronic disease. Previously, HBV genotypes have been classified into eight genotypes (A-H) and because of genome diversity is a hallmark of HBV virus allowed its classification into (10) genotypes (A–J). The clinical relevance of such genotype is yet unclear. Detection of HBV genotype is very important to clarify the pathogenesis, rout of infection and virulence of the virus. The major classification of HBV subtype is sorted into 4 subtypes or serotypes (*adr*, *adw*, *ayr*, and *ayw*). The four possible combinations define the major subtypes and additional amino acids contribute to immunogenicity. These subtypes can be further classified into (9) serotypes (adw2, adw4q-, adrq+, adrq-, ayw1, ayw2, ayw3, ayw4 and ayr). Epidemiologic studies found that the prevalence of these serotypes varies in different parts of the world.

Keywords: HBV, genotype, serotype, subtype, *Hepadnaviridae*

1. Introduction

Hepatitis simply means inflammation of liver. This word came from heap: the Latin for liver and "titis" means inflammation. In addition to viruses, many varieties of agents can cause hepatitis such as bacteria, parasites, fungi and chemical agents including drugs, toxins and alcohol [1, 2].

Currently, 11 types of viruses are recognize causing hepatitis, Epstein- Barr virus (EBV), Cytomegalovirus (CMV) and 9 of hepatotropic viruses. Only 3 out of these 9 viruses are well characterized from A-E. Hepatitis A (HAV) sometimes called infectious hepatitis. Hepatitis B (HBV) is called serum hepatitis. Hepatitis C (formerly none A or B hepatitis NABA). Hepatitis D (HDV) which is formerly enteric transmitted hepatitis. Newly discovered forms of viral hepatitis including hepatitis F (HFV), hepatitis G (HGV), Transfusion Transmitted virus (TTV) and SEN virus. They all predominantly affect and infect liver cells. Despite significant overlap in the clinical manifestation caused by them, these types of viruses differ widely in their morphology, genomic organization, taxonomic classification and mode of replication [2–4].

Hepatitis B infection is a global health problem which is 50–100 times more infectious than HIV. Approximately 400 million people are carriers of chronic liver disease every year due to consequences of the disease [5–7]. Not only HBV can infect hepatocytes but also infects in extrahepatic sites including lymph nodes, bone marrow, circulating lymphocytes, spleen and pancreas. Hepatitis B virus can occur as an acute or chronic disease [8].

People at high risk of infection including those requiring frequent transfusions or hemodialysis, physicians, dentists, nurses, and other health care workers, intravenous drug users, police, firemen and others who are likely to come into contact with potentially infected blood products [9], as well as, sexual contacts with an acute or chronically infected persons. In the US, homosexually active men consist of 6%, whereas heterosexually with multiple partners consist of 0.5% from all risk factors [10].

Approximately 5% of the infected world's population may lead to cirrhosis and HCC worldwide. It is approximated that (500, 000 to 1000, 000) persons die annually from HBV related liver disease. Most infections occur at birth or during early childhood. Infections usually cluster in households of chronically infected patients [11].

2. Acute hepatitis B

Acute disease typically occurs in the infected adolescents or adult who have not been vaccinated. This acute presentation can be life threatening due to massive liver damage from the host immune reactions [12]. Most people with HBV experience few or no symptoms; in fact, a 65% are unaware that they carry the virus. Although, a 30% of people with acute hepatitis B have no symptoms and most people with chronic HBV also have few or no symptoms, most symptoms may include fatigue (unusual, prolonged tiredness), fever, malaise (a flu-like feeling), nausea, vomiting,

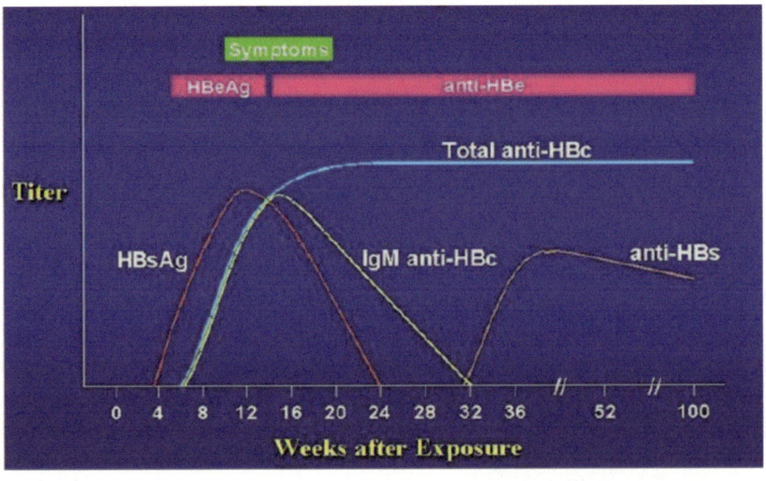

Figure 1.
Acute hepatitis B virus infection with recovery typical serological course. http://virology-online.com/viruses/index.htm.

yellowing of skin and eyes (Jaundice), loss of appetite (anorexia), abdominal pain or bloating, indigestion, headache, itching (pruritus) and muscles or joints aches [13]. Acute hepatitis may in some cases progress to fulminant hepatitis leading to liver failure, which is a state with high mortality [6]. The weak immune response generated by young children acutely infected hepatocytes. For this reason, clinical symptoms suggestive of acute HBV infection are frequently absent in this patients population. For those patients who resolve their infection, HBsAg disappears at about 3–6 month, often just prior to the detection of antibodies to hepatitis B surface antigen (anti-HBs), while some patients with self-limited infection, however may still have low levels of HBV DNA in blood; whether the HBV DNA is a part of intact virions remains unknown [14].

In some people, the hepatitis B virus can also cause a chronic liver infection that can later develop into cirrhosis (a scarring of the liver) or liver cancer (http://virology-online.com/viruses/HepatitisB.htm) (**Figure 1**).

3. Chronic hepatitis B

Chronic HBV (CHB) infection can be define as the presence of hepatitis B surface antigen (HBsAg) in the serum of an infected individuals for at least six months or as the presence of HBsAg in a patient who is negative for immunoglobulin M antibodies to the hepatitis B core antigen (anti-HBc).

Chronic hepatitis can be divided into four stages. The first stage, the immune tolerance phase which is characterized by active viral replication and immune system tolerance. In this initial phase, HBV DNA replicates at a high levels and the HBsAg and HBeAg can be detectable while the Aminotransferase (ALT) levels are normal or low, mild or no liver necroinflamation and no or slow progression of fibrosis. In this phase, more prolonged in subjects infected prenatally or in the first years of life. Next, the immune clearance phase: The immunologic response is causing inflammation and hepatic injury as a result of viral clearance. Here, the ALT levels are elevated and moderate/severe necroinflammation in liver biopsy is observed. The third phase, inactive carrier state: The viral clearance is accompanied by seroconversion of HBsAg, resulting in relatively low HBV DNA level and normalized ALT levels. Few patients reach the final stage, when the HBsAg is

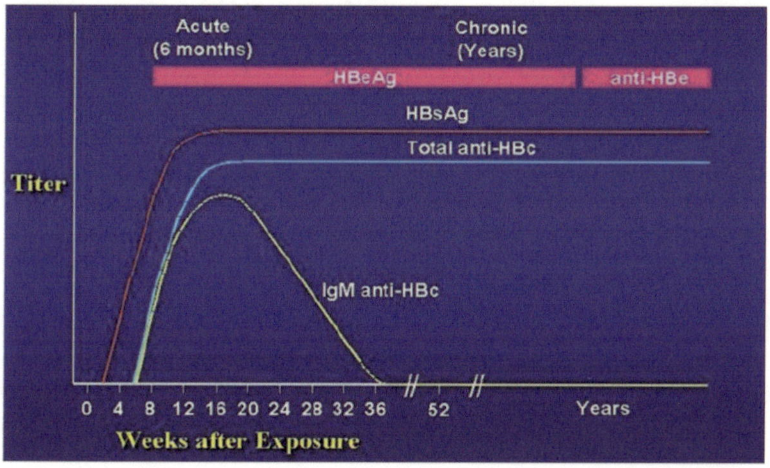

Figure 2.
Progression of chronic hepatitis B virus infection typical serological course. http://virology-online.com/viruses/index.htm.

completely cleared and anti-HBs becomes detectable as a sign of immunity [6, 13, 15]. The risk of developing chronic hepatitis B infection that depends on the age at which infection is acquired. The risk is the lowest in adults and > 90% in neonates whose mothers are HBeAg-positive. Chronic infection is less frequent in those infected as the children. The risk of becoming chronically infected with hepatitis B is increased in those whose immunity is impaired [16]. Clinically, the e-antigen HBeAg is important in chronic infection as it is regarded a marker for replication and indicative of ongoing infection. When seroconversion occurs, it normally reflects remission of liver disease and viral clearance [6]. Persons with chronic HBV may have HBeAg or anti-HBe in their sera. In persons who are HBeAg positive, spontaneous seroconversion from HBeAg to anti-HBe commonly occurs with often accompanied by a flare in aminotransferase ALT levels. After conversion of HBeAg to anti-HBe, most persons have normal ALT levels and lower levels of HBV DNA which is usually $<10^3$ copies / ml (**Figure 2**) [17].

4. Occult hepatitis B infection (OBI)

In this stage of infection, HBV DNA in the serum or in the liver may in some cases still be detectable in the absence of HBsAg which is termed occult hepatitis B. The clinical importance of this is not completely understood, but occult hepatitis B has been associated with reactivation in the setting of immunosuppression and enhancing risk for liver cancer [6, 18]. This type of infection represents a potential transmission source of HBV via blood transfusion or organ transplantation. In addition, occult HBV infection has been associated with cryptogenic CH and HCC. Furthermore, some studies suggested that occult hepatitis B might affect responsiveness of chronic HCV to interferon therapy and disease progress [9].

5. Cirrhosis and hepatocellular carcinoma (HCC)

Some reports have been estimated that up to 40% of individuals with chronic hepatitis B (CHB) will progress to cirrhosis [13, 19, 20] and may lead to hepatocellular carcinoma (HCC). Worldwide, more than 50% of HCC cases, and in highly endemic areas 70–80% of HCC cases are attributable to HBV and 20% of the 400 million people with chronic hepatitis B infection will develop to HCC. It has been showed that the presence of HBeAg and higher levels of HBV DNA have been found to be strong risk factors for HCC in patients with chronic HBV infection and mainly develops in patients with liver cirrhosis [6, 19, 21]. The mechanisms of oncogenesis by HBV remain obscure. HBV may stimulate active regeneration and cirrhosis which may be associated with long-term chronicity. However, HBV associates tumors occasionally arise in the absence of cirrhosis, and such hypotheses do not explain the frequent finding of integrated viral DNA in tumors. Although insertional mutagenesis of HBV remains an attractive hypothesis to explain its oncogenicity. Like many other cancers, there is insufficient supportive evidence development of hepatocellular carcinoma likely to be a multifactorial process [22]. The incidence of HCC may also be affected by factors other than HBV infection such as HCV co-infection, alcohol intake and aflatoxin B1 in the food supply. In the Amazonian basin, the genotype F infections are associated with fulminant hepatitis, but this occurs in the context of co-infection or super infection with Hepatitis Delta Virus (HDV) genotype III [17, 23].

Many other risk factors have been implicated in the progression of liver disease and the development of HCC. In such co-infections have been reported that HBV may carriers with more than one genotype. Some common co- infection occurs

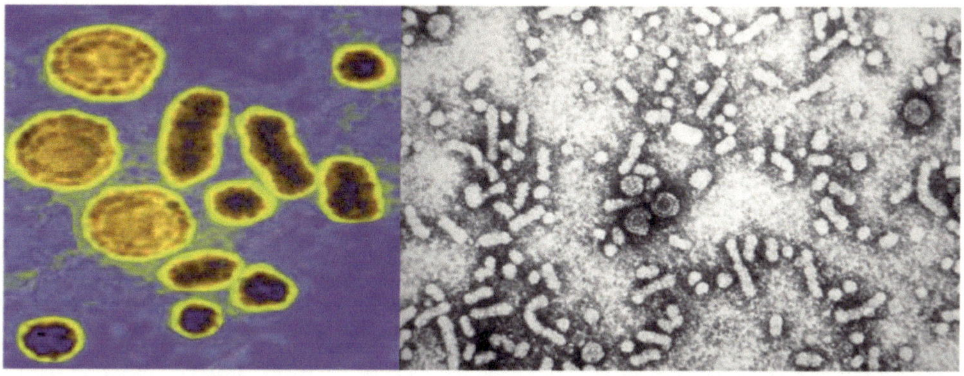

Figure 3.
EM of HBV particles, https://www.google.com/search?source=univ&tbm=isch&q=hepatitis+B+virus+electron+microscope+images&client=opera&sa=X&ved=2ahUKEwiTsoLLsajwAhVSNOwKHXCvCuoQjJkEegQIAxAB&biw=1366&bih=658.

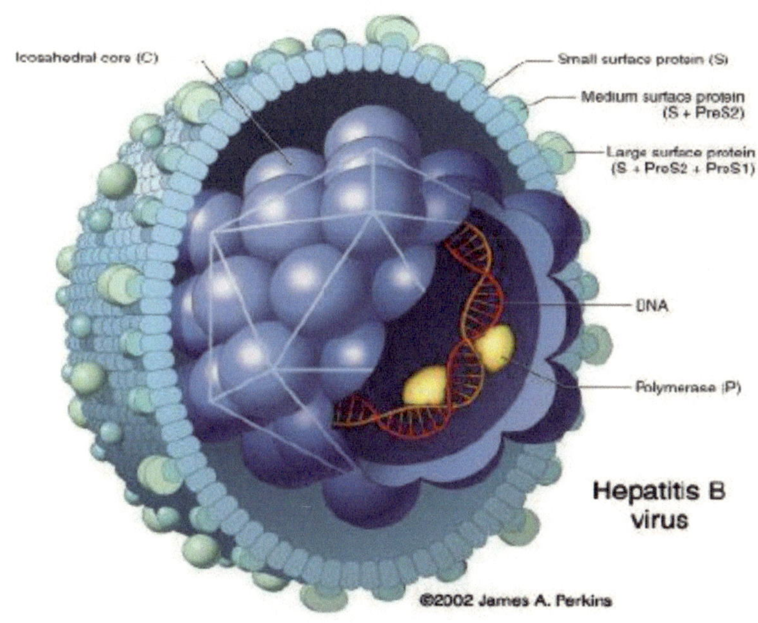

Figure 4.
The architecture of a Dane particle. https://people.rit.edu/japfaa/infectious.html.

between genotype B and C, A and D, which is presumably due to the coexistence of these genotypes in the same regions. Recombination between genotypes has been reported as genotypes A with D [24]. The clinical impact of co-infections is unclear, but the viral loads have been reported to be higher in the co-infected patients. The frequency of co- infection may be associated with genotyping method as the reported frequency varies widely [6]. Persons who are co-infected with both HBV and HCV also have an increased risk of developing HCC, as compared with those who are infected with either virus alone. Even though, co-infection with HDV has not been shown to increase the risk of HCC. One study demonstrated that HCC appears at younger ages in co-infected persons than it does in those infected solely with HBV. Using chronic alcohol also appears to increase the risk of cirrhosis (**Figures 3** and **4**) [17].

6. HBV genotypes

The clinical relevance of such genotype is yet unclear. However, because the HBV induced disease is the resultant of virus-host interaction, the disease characteristics may be influenced by the genotypes of the virus [5]. HBV genotype and subgenotype are strong factors in predicting outcomes of chronic HBV infections [25].

Traditionally, HBV genotypes has been based on one of the following criteria: an intergroup divergence of 8% (similarity in 92%) [26, 27] or greater over the complete genome sequence, or 4 ± 1% or greater divergence of the surface antigen HBsAg [28]. Detection of HBV genotype is very important to clarify the pathogenesis, rout of infection and virulence of the virus [29]. In the context of the findings described, there might be a need to further differentiate between genetic variants versus genotypes [30]. Since the HBV genotype is due to the entire nucleotide sequence, the HBV genotype is more appropriate for investigation of geographic distribution and epidemiologic connections [31]. Previously, HBV genotypes have been classified into eight genotypes (A-H) and because of genome diversity is a hallmark of HBV virus allowed its classification into (10) genotypes (A–J) [32, 33]. Genotypes A-D were identified in 1988 under the sequence divergence in the entire genome exceeding 8%, and designated by capital letters of the alphabet [34]. Genotype E-F were identified in 1993 and genotype G was identified in 2000. Genotype H which is phylogenetically closely related to genotype F was proposed in 2002 [6]. Genotype I has been described and isolated from Hanoi in the northern part of Vietnam, Laos, a primitive tribe from northeast India as well as in the northwest of China [18, 35, 36]. Finally, the newest genotype J was identified in the Ryukyu Islands in Japan and this genotype has a close relationship with gibbon/orangutan genotypes, and human genotype C [37].

Zekri and coworkers found that HBV mixed genotype infections could probably be of clinical significance in HBV-induced liver diseases. He established that prevalence of mixed A/D genotype infections related to induce chronic liver diseases and evaluation of therapy [38].

6.1 Relationship between HBV genotypes

There are structural, functional, infectivity and clinical differences between HBV genotypes. Such differences include prognosis, progression of disease, complications as cirrhosis and hepatocellular carcinoma, as well as response to antiviral therapy. Structurally, HBV genotypes differ in the length of their genomes. The numbering of HBV genome from the EcoRI site leads to difficulties in comparing nucleotide

Genotype	Length	Insertion/Depletion
A	3221	Insertion core: 6 bp
B	3215	
C	3215	
D	3182	Depletion Pre-S1: 33 bp
E	3212	Depletion Pre-S1: 3 bp
F	3215	
G	3248	Insertion core: 36 bp, Depletion Pre-S1: 3 bp
H	3215	

Table 1.
Differences between the main HBV genotypes [6].

positions between genotypes. Functionally, the Pre-S region that is important for virus attachment and cell entry, shows momentous differences between genotypes. Genotype A differs mainly in sequence of the Pre-S2 region, and has insertion of six nucleotides in the terminal protein portion of the polymerase gene overlapping the core gene, and shares some structural features with genotype F. Genotype D genome is most similar to Genotype E, especially in the X-gene. Differences in RNA splicing folding between genotypes could be predicted [39].

A recent study by Chan et al. indicated that genotype C was associated with more severe liver fibrosis than genotype B probably because of delayed HBeAg sero-conversion and prolonged active disease [20, 40]. The major structural differences between HBV genotypes are shown in **Table 1** (2.1) below depending on nucleotide numbering, length and characteristic indels of HBV genotypes:

7. Prevalence and epidemiology of genotypes and subgenotypes

Humans are only reservoir for HBV, which is 50–100 times more infectious than HIV. The prevalence of HBV infection varies in different parts of the world, with most of the disease burden occurring in Asia and Africa [41].

8. Genotype A

Genotype A derived mainly from Europe, India, Africa, and North America [42]. The existence of subgenotypes within genotype A has been reported (A1/Aa) from South Africa and South Asia. Subgenotype Ae/A2 is mainly endemic in Europe and United States. Ac/A3 is mostly found among populations of West and Central Africa [21]. These subgenotypes were significantly distinguished by bootstrap at phylogenetic analyses complete genomes. The differences between European and Afro-Asian of genotype A strains that the subgenotype A1 strains encoding Asn (207) and Leu (209), while the A2 strains had Ser (207) and Val (209). All strains specifying ayw1 serotype belonged to A1, and most of them were from Africa. Genotype A is corresponding to subtype adw [8, 42].

8.1 Genotype A and its subgenotypes

Genotype A is distinguished at the carboxylic end of the core gene by a 6 nucleotide insert. A comprehensive analytical study of genotype A led to classification of A1, A2, A4, and A3 subgenotype, as the latter sequence category did not follow the subgenotype classification criterion. The subgenotypes A1, A4 and A3 are mostly present in Africa, while A2 prevails in Northern, Central and Northern Europe and in North America [8, 42].

9. Genotype B

Genotype B is originated mainly from China, Japan, and Southeast Asia (Vietnam, Thailand, and Indonesia). Four subgenotypes, designated B1–B4, were confirmed by significant bootstrap when comparing complete genomes [24, 42]. Other classification of genotype B isolates into two groups: Bj ("j" stands for Japan), mostly found in Japan, and Ba ("a" stands for Asia) [43]. All strains specified adw2 serotype with the exception of the strains in B4 which specified ayw1 or adw3 serotype according to the strain. Subgenotype B1 was formed mainly by 18 of the

25 S genes of genotype B strains from Japan, corresponding to the described group Bj while the most genotype B strains from China belonged to subgenotype B2 which also comprised strains from Vietnam. Subgenotype B3 was formed by four strains from Indonesia. Subgenotype B4 comprised only strains from Vietnam. Apart from the Arg (122) in B4, there were no amino acid substitutions in HBsAg characteristic of individual subgenotypes within B [42].

9.1 Novel subgenotypes of genotype B

The subgenotypes of B have been reclassified into six subgenotypes, namely: B1, B2, B4–B6 and quasi-subgenotype B3 according to the new classification with a phylogenetic and sequence divergence of >4 percent. In contrast to the remaining subgenotypes of B that have this mixture, subgenotype B1 (previously Bj), found in mainly Japan and B5 (previously B6) from the Canadian Inuit population, are genotype B without recombination with Genotype C in the precore/core area. Subgene B1 was presumably B5's ancestor, likely transported from Siberia and Alaska to North America and Greenland by indigenous peoples during the migration [42].

10. Genotype C

Genotype C genome shows four subgenotypes, C1–C4 [21] supported by 96–100% bootstrap with clear geographical clustering. The ayr subtype is widespread in genotype C. Australian strains specified ayw3. In the subgenotypes C1–C3, there were an intermixture within the adr strains of strains specifying adw2 or ayr. The constraints against substitutions of subtype specifying residues122 and 160 thus seem less pronounced for genotype C than for the other genotypes. C1 was formed by the majority of the strains from the Far East (Japan, Korea, and China) [42]. Sakamoto found a novel subgenotypes of HBV/C5 and HBV/B5 among chronic liver disease patients in the Philippines [44].

10.1 Novel subgenotypes of genotype C

Genetic C is the earliest HBV genotype, according to Paraskevis et al. The C1–C16, which represents a longer period of endemicity in humans, is the largest number of subgenotypes. In Indonesia, there are a significant number of sub-genotypes. Subgenotype C4 is solely present in northern Australian aboriginal people that came down from a group of establishments who emigrated at least 50.000 years ago from Africa [44].

10.2 Genotype D

Genotype D is the most widespread genotype and predominated in the Mediterranean area, the Near East, and as far as India. It was also found in Aboriginal populations in Asia from Indonesia and Papua. The strains specified ayw2, ayw3, or ayw4 serotype with the exception of two European strain specifying Lys (122), Thr (127), and Lys (160) corresponding to the putative subtype adw3. Phylogenetic analysis of complete genomes have been distinguishing four subgenotypes D1–D4. Strains specifying ayw2 were found in D1, D3, and D4. The geographical distribution of the subgenotypes within D was less restricted than that of genotypes A, B, and C. Although, the strains from Middle East mainly belonged to D1 [25] those from South Africa and Alaska mainly to D3, while those from Oceania and Somalia were only found in D4 [42]. Genotype D is currently segregated into eight subgenotypes (D1–D8). A novel D9 isolates do not possess any unique motif in the Pre-S/S ORF that can distinguish them from the other eight subgenotypes of D. D9 subgenotype is originated from discrete recombination events between genotypes D and C as evident from the fact that both genotype C and D9 sequences are monophyletic in the core region [32]. Genotype D is characterized by a 33 nucleotide deletion at the N-terminus of the Pre-S1 region, therefore it has the shortest genome of the eight HBV genotypes (3182 nucleotides) [18].

11. Novel information of genotype D

In an analysis of the subgenotypes of D recently, it has been concluded that there are six, not eight subgenotypes. Subgenotypes D1–D6 can be distinguished by a separate cluster with high bootstrap support and amino acid signature. Subgenotype D3 and subgenotype D6 were reclassified as one sub-genotype D3, and genotype D/E instead of subgenotype was found to be genotype D/E. The D4 subgenottom may be an early substratum of early human intercontinental migration and may occur in indigenous peoples in Papua New Guinea and Australia and in a limited proportion of the Canadian Inuit people. In addition, a subgenotype D4 recombinant was same [18].

12. Genotype E

Genotype E is definitely the dominant genotype in West Africa and has very low intra-genotypic diversity suggesting that this genotype has spread only recently [21]. Genotype E strains specified of subtype ayw4, and all derived from West Africa apart from one strain which was derived from Madagascar. There were no subdivisions or specific amino acid substitutions distinguishing the strains from each other. All strains expressed Ser (140) also present in the genotype F. Study analysis of the complete genome of genotype E strains showed that the chimpanzee strain was not ancestral as compared with the human strains. This chimpanzee has probably also been inoculated with human serum at capture, since the majority of indigenous HBV strains from chimpanzees cluster separately from human strains [42].

Genotype E has the single Ayw 4 serologic subtype, which can be separated from A–D, F, H and I by the preS1 region's deletion of 3 nucleotides. In West, Central Africa this genotype is endemic to a poor genetic diversity which has led to the recent appearance of more than 200 years. Contrary to the slavic trading subgenotype A1, genotype E is scarcely present outside Africa, with the exception of persons of African origin who further affirm its recently emerging after forced slavery migrations. A median developmental period of 130 years has been estimated using Bayesian inference, from the most recent common ancestor (tMRCA), this varies from a tMRCA predicted by others for 6,000 years. However, as previously indicated, genotype E may have occurred and recently been reintroduced in indigenous African populations. In persons with no experience of traveling to or from Africa, genotype E isolated from Pygmies and Khoi San, and in Colombia and India. The variation of the predicted genotype E age would be difficult to overcome without a precise determination of the nucleotide HBV substitution rate [42].

13. Genotype F

Genotype F has been isolated from Amerindian population in different countries [21]. Genotype F strains are subdivided into four subgenotypes. Subgenotype F1 particular F1a have been found in Alaska, El - Salvador, Guatemala, Costa Rica and Nicaragua; whereas F1b has been reported in Peru and Argentina. Strains of subgenotype F2 has been found in Costa Rica, Nicaragua, Venezuela and Brazil. Subgenoype F3 is found in Colombia and Venezuela and F4 in Bolivia and Argentina [21]. F1 and F2, each characterized by specific substitutions in the S gene product, Leu (45) and Thr (45), respectively. Subgenotype F1 was mainly formed by strains from Central America. F2 mainly containing strains from South America encompassed all strains from Venezuela and Colombia and the few strains from Polynesia and were characterized by an Asp (2) Glu substitution. Subtype adw4q– is alongside with adrq– the dominating subtypes in Polynesia. This supports a dual origin of its population, and the close relation of the Polynesian strain to strains from Colombia. Most of genotype F strains specified adw4 subtype. All had the Pro (178) Gln substitution assumed to abolish the expression of q. Some strains lacked the Pro (127) Leu substitution characteristic of genotype F and specified the putative subtype adw2q [42].

14. Genotype G

Genotype G is mostly detected in co-infection with other HBV genotypes with mostly genotype A [21]. Genotype G strains are originating from the USA, Mexico, and Europe [6] which are all specifying adw2 subtype. The genotype G strains shared two unique substitutions, Gln (51) Leu and Thr (63) Ile, were not found in any other genotype. The S gene products of the strains showed the highest similarity to those of genotype A. However, these strains showed a high divergence from the other HBV strains, when complete genomes were compared [42]. Genotype G strains have a 36 bp insertion immediately after the initiation codon of the C gene, increasing the size of HBcAg by (12 aa). This does not effect on Polymerase but a one codon deletion in the Pre-S1 region reduces both Pre-S1 and Pol by one aa [23].

Genotype G is characterized by the use, at the positions 2 and 28 in the precore/core region, of a 3′ nucleotide insert, 3′ of position 1905 and two translation stop codons which abrogate HBeAg. Only in the presence of other genotypes, most often genotype A, that may supply HBeAg in Trans, may chronic infection be identified. Sexual reproduction by males who have sex with men is a significant risk factor. Genotype G is not as diverse from genotype E with which the deletion of 3-nucleotide occurs in the central area and a special preS sequence. Since the African root of genotype G was not yet found in Africa [23].

15. Genotype H

All strains belonging to the genotype H derived from Nicaragua, Mexico, and California. These strains differ from genotype F strains by two unique substitutions, Val (144) and Pro (45), as well as Ile (57),Thr (140), Phe (158), and Ala (224) [42, 45, 46].

16. Genotype I and its subgenotypes

In 2008, a study sequence of the whole genome (AB231908) of the Vietnamese male was suggested that it was closely linked to three previously identified Vietnamese 'aberrant' strains as well as to one of the 9th, I genotype. This was unacceptable since the average genetic divergence of these 4 genotype C strains was 7%, and the recombination study was not strong. The following sequences is derived from Laos, the tribe of the Idu Mishmi in North-East India, Canadian of Vietnamese origin, and China. At least 7.5 per cent of the nucleotide divergence between each of these sequences was with strong group bootstrap assistance, thus satisfying the genotype assignment criterion. Two subgenotypes I1 and I2, respectively, were identified with serological subtype's adw 2 and ayw 2. This subgenotype isolation was challenged by the sequencing of additional Indian cluster strains in subgenotype I2 and by an estimated intersubgenotype differences of <4%. The intergroup divergences between subgenotype I1 and I2 were found to be 3,40 ± 0,30 percent (mean ± SD) below the 4 percent cut, if we analyzed all 19 genotype I genomes without indels in the GenBank. However, an exception should be made for subgenotype D1 and D2 due to the distinct serological subtypes. 4.1% between Laotian strain FJ023663 and the Indian strain EU835242 were the largest intergroup divergence. This genotype is endemic in a broad region of Asia for a long time because of the extensive geographical range. Genotype I is a recombinant of A/C/G genotypes and an indeterminate genotype which, when analyzed, is closely related to C genotype and the genotype A of polymerase genotype. The areas of genotype A and C are closely associated with A3s and C3s. In both Huh7 cells and acute hydrodynamic mouse infection, Genotype I has been functionally characterized. The two schemes also secreted genotype I at levels comparable to genotype A, genotype B and generic C and higher than generic D, but genotype A at levels related to genotype A and below B, C and D [42, 45, 46].

17. Genotype J

This strain had been isolated from one Japanese man who had long-term residence in Borneo with hepatocellular carcinoma (HCC). The entire non-human HBV genome clusters including gibbon isolates, orangutans, chimpanzees and gorillas. Their rates diverged 10.7–15.7% from other genotypes relative to 1,440 human and non-human HBV strains and did not demonstrate any indication that they were recombined. In the later study, Locarnini et al. concluded that genotype 'J' is actually a recombinant of genotype C and gibbon HBV in the S area, using additionally the gibbon/orangutan sequences for contrast. Therefore, while there is a strong

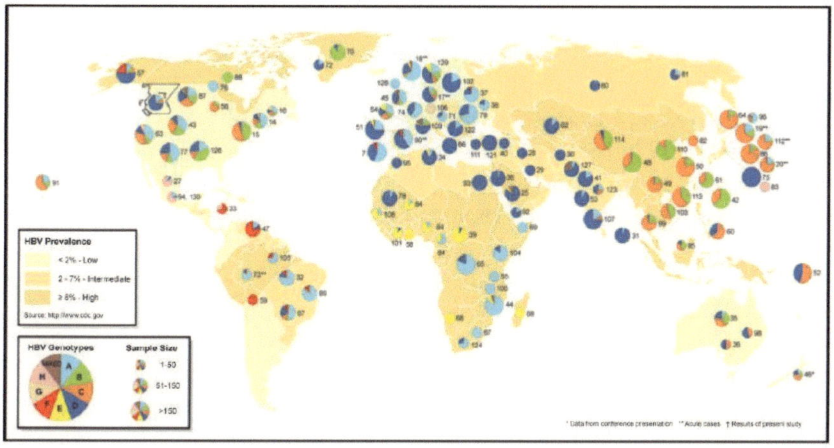

Figure 5.
Global geographical distribution of HBV genotypes. https://www.ncbi.nlm.nih.gov/pmc/articles/PMC4969325/pdf/40506_2016_Article_80.pdf.

intergroup divergency of genotype J, this will reflect propagation of cross species, detection and examination of additional sequences, until the presence of this last genotype can be verified. This requirement is defined for classification into separate genotype (**Figure 5**) [18].

Some studies have shown that different HBV genotypes and subgenotypes may cause differences in disease progression, response to antiviral treatment regimens and in clinical outcomes. Therefore, the accurate classification of HBV is important for clinical and etiological investigations [47].

18. HBV serotypes

The major classification of HBV subtype is sorted into 4 subtypes or serotypes (adr, adw, ayr, and ayw) [21, 45]. The molecular basis for this classification was variation at few sites in the S region. The 'a' determinant (aa 124–148) is the major antigenic determinant common and confers protection against all serotypes [41], while the d/y and w/r variations depend on Lys/Arg substitutions at residue (122) and (160) respectively [6]. If the amino acid at position (122) is Arg (122R) then the subtype is y, and if it is Lys (122 K) then the subtype is d. In the same way, (160R) defines the r subtype and (160 K) defines the w subtype. The four possible combinations define the major subtypes and additional amino acids contribute to immunogenicity. These subtypes can be further classified into (9) serotypes (adw2, adw4q-, adrq+, adrq-, ayw1, ayw2, ayw3, ayw4 and ayr). Epidemiologic studies found that the prevalence of these serotypes varies in different parts of the world. To date, there has been very little data on the clinical significance of HBV serotypes [45]. While the ability to detect HBsAg was of obvious importance for the safety of the blood supply, serotyping was useful for widely employed in clinical, virological, epidemiological studies, including studies of nosocomial and iatrogenic infections and intra-familial transmission, [23, 48].

Determinants w1/w2, w3 and w4 are classified by Pro, Thr or Leu substitutions at residue (127) respectively. w1 variation is distinguished by Arg122, Phe134 and/or Ala159 [49]. It has been found that the epitope in adw contains (18Val-19Pro), whereas these amino acids are replaced by hydrophilic residues Thr-Ser in the ayw1, 2, and 3 subtypes. As a consequence of these substitutions, the conformation of the epitopes, as predicted by 3D modeling and analysis of crystal structures, was drastically changed [50]. Cui and coworkers found that the serotype adw is based on Lys (120) and Lys (160). To a large extent, genotypes and subgenotypes have replaced the usage of serotypes. Most ayw serotypes are grouped in genotypes B and D [51]. The serotype ayw occurs in all genotypes except in 'C'. Serotype adw is associated with all genotypes except D and E, whereas adr and ayr subtypes are encountered with genotype C [5]. There is no stringent correlation between phenotypic HBsAg markers and sequence variation outside the S gene but such a correlation between genetic and phenotypic markers is required for epidemiological studies [52].

19. Detect HBV genotype

Detection of HBV genotype is very important to clarify the pathogenesis, rout of infection and virulence of the virus. The HBV genotypes are variable that could potentially influence the outcome of chronic HBV and the success of antiviral therapy. HBV genotype testing has not yet been widely adopted in clinical laboratories. A variety of methods have been used, including whole or partial genome sequencing, PCR based restriction fragment length polymorphism (RFLP), genotype-specific PCR amplification, PCR plus hybridization, line probe assay, enzyme-linked immunoassay and serology. Whole-genome sequencing is the "gold standard," and it is particularly accurate for detecting recombinant viruses [38, 53]. The common assays are:

19.1 INNO-LiPA

This reverse hybridization method has been developed by Innogenetics and is commercially available as INNO-LiPA. This method is easy to perform, very convenient, rapid method [54, 55], and suitable for detecting mixed genotype infections. First, HBV DNA is amplified by PCR using biotinylated primers complementary to a conserved sequence in the S/Pre-S ORF. The amplified biotinylated PCR products are then hybridized to probes immobilized onto membrane strips that detect genotype specific differences in the HBV polymerase gene domains B to C. After washing, alkaline phosphatase (ALP) - labeled streptavidin is added, followed by substrate (BCIP/NBT chromogen) that gives a purple/brown precipitate in the presence of ALP. The overall success rate is 98% [56]. These methods may fail to type all isolates and interpretation of results may be difficult particularly in the case of mixed genotype infections [55]. In addition, this assay is not suitable for large- scale surveys nor accurate to identify mixed infection [57].

19.2 HBV DNA-Chip assay

The whole HBV genome is amplified by a duplex PCR. The labeled PCR products were purified using a purification kit. Samples were hybridized on the HBV DNA-Chip prototype and stained with streptavidin-phycoerythrin conjugate on a GeneChip fluidics station 400. Finally, the HBV DNA-Chips were scanned on an HP Gene Array scanner and were analyzed by using DNA-Chip evaluation software. DNA-Chip technology is currently not used routinely in a clinical laboratory [58].

19.3 Nested-multiplex qPCR

A detection assay is used specific primers. This assay is greater accuracy in genotyping and greater sensitivity to identify mixed genotypes when compared to sequencing reactions. This method can be useful with large clinical scale and epidemiological studies, especially in regions with high prevalence of HBV infection [59].

19.4 Oligonucleotide microarray

Can determine genotypes A-G. The amplified products are heat-denatured and added to silylated slides, to which genotype-specific probes are immobilized [56].

19.5 Enzyme immunoassay (EIA)

This commercially assay is used with monoclonal antibodies raised against genotype specific epitopes in the Pre-S2. Although this assay may fail to type the HBV DNA in clinical samples due to the presence of mixtures of genotypes or low levels of HBsAg in the sample, it offers a convenient, serologically based assay, [55, 60]. EIAs were less sensitive than rapid assays [61]. ELISAs for HBsAg are generally considered more sensitive. It has been showed that the samples with low HBsAg/HBcAg ratios were much more likely to have undetectable Pre-S2 epitopes by the genotyping ELISA that used [31].

19.6 TaqMan-MGB probe

This assay has several advantages. On the one hand, conjugated MGB can improve the melting temperature of probe, thus increasing probe specificity. In addition, it permits shorter probes to be used (usually 13 to 18 nt). On the other hand, shorter probes make fluorescence and quencher closer A type-specific nested PCR assay established and applied for investigation of HBV genotype. The TaqMan technique is suitable for typing [40, 62, 63].

19.7 Line probe assay

This assay is detected sequence specific oligomers for each genotype are immortalized on a paper strip, to which PCR amplified test samples are hybridized (reverse hybridization) [5].

20. Limitations of using in-house assays

Many of limitations emerge when using in-house assays depending on the type of assay. It has often been suggested that in-house PCR assays suffer from problems with standardization, false positivity, or contamination, making them unsuitable for routine clinical diagnostic use [58]. The lack of an internal control does not allow to rule out false-negative results due to the presence of inhibitors to PCR amplification. The limit of detection and the upper limit of the dynamic range are approximates, as a lot more replicates and lot-to- lot testing would be necessary to verify these values.

One disadvantage of ELISA is that not all antibodies can be used monoclonal antibodies must be qualified as matched pairs, meaning they must recognize separate epitopes on the antigen so they do not hinder each other's binding. Also, there is a limit to its sensitivity since the amplification is restricted by the amount of enzyme that can be conjugated to antibodies. Immunoreactivity of the antibody may be reduced by enzyme labeling, which in itself is an expensive and time-consuming process [64].

HBV genotyping based on complete genome sequences is an ideal methods, but sequencing is still expensive and not easy to carry out for large scale study. The developed precise PCR genotyping system using type-specific primers, allowing the identification of types A through F. This assay system may be useful for rapid and sensitive genotyping of the HBV genome either epidemiological, pathological, transmission studies and can be carried out in large scale. Mixed-genotype infection is very difficult to detect by direct sequencing. Since direct sequencing or Sanger sequencing can pick up mixed populations only at ratios above 20:80 simultaneous [24, 40, 47, 60, 65, 66].

20.1 PCR-RFLP

RFLP depends usually on PCR amplification of the S gene, restriction enzyme digestion, and separation of digested fragments by electrophoresis. A combination of different restriction enzymes has been used for RFLP, the choice of which has been determined according to the different HBV genotype sequences in GenBank. This method has been used to determine genotypes A–F. In 2004, Zeng et al. developed a modified RFLP technique based on the S gene allowing the detection of HBV genotypes A–H. In this method, two PCR rounds were undertaken prior to restriction enzyme digestion by five enzymes, namely StyI, BsrI, DpnI, HpaII, and EaeI. The method was compared with another RFLP method targeting the Pre-S1 region and the results were concordant in 96.8% [54].

RFLP typically relies on Sgene enhancement PCR, restrictive digestion of the enzyme, and electrophoresis isolation of the digested fragments. RFLP was used for a mixture of various restrictive enzymes, which were determined by the different HBV genotype sequences in GenBank. This approach is used in the A–F genotype determination. In 2004, Zeng et al. introduced a modified S-based RFLP technique that detects HBV A–H genotypes. In this process, five enzymes, StyI, BsrI, DpnI, Hpaii and EaeI, were used before the restriction of enzyme digestion. The method was contrasted with another RFLP method for the Pre-S1 field, with 96, 8 percent of the data.

Nested PCR-RFLP method for HBV genotyping is simple and inexpensive for clinical diagnostic in large scale. PCR-RFLP assay is more sensitive to identifying HBV viral populations [28]. This method can detect mixed genotypes and can determine subgenotypes in large population studies [56]. Toan et al. used the restriction enzyme Tsp509I to restrict patterns and predicted fragment sizes determined HBV genotypes, while Zeng et al. used five restriction enzymes, StyI, BsrI, DpnI, HpaII and EaeI were deemed to be suitable for yielding restriction patterns. These enzymes restrict at Per-S region (other study used EcoR1. This novel method would identify several relative advantages. Firstly, it can identify all eight HBV genotypes. Secondly, it is more accurate because it was based on analyzing many of the sequences deposited in GeneBank. Thirdly, a simple and inexpensive strategy can be adopted according to the most prevalent HBV genotypes in a particular geographical region. Moreover, this method can be useful in evaluating clinical, epidemiological and virological differences between genotypes [67]. Venegas used restriction enzymes Sau3A I, Bsr I or Hpa II to cut the DNA at S region. Vivekanandan and coworkers were used HinfI and Tsp 509I restriction enzymes but he found that genotypes could not be assigned for a small proportion of strains and this may be due to the presence of infection with multiple genotypes or with strains that have altered and or additional recognition sites for the restriction enzymes used in testing [68]. Neisi et al. used AvaII and mboI restriction enzymes but he resulted that the RFLP method cannot type mixed genotype infections. Other study used AvaII and DpnII [69, 70].

Badar used five restriction enzymes AlwI, EarI, HphI, NciI and NlaIV. He explained that the genotyping system can help to evaluate the etiological or clinical relevance of HBV genotypes and to predict the progression of liver disease or to investigate routes of infection [67]. Allen and coworkers described that the RFLP assay method has been commonly used for identifying known polymorphisms in DNA from many organisms or tissues and for detecting YMDD motif variations associated with in vitro lamivudine resistance patients. Moreover, although the RFLP assay was more sensitive in identifying HBV viral populations, one advantage of DNA sequencing over the RFLP that the DNA sequence provides information at sites other than at specific codons and continues to be useful in the detection of sequence variations at other sites for detecting quasi species. PCR-RFLP has some limitations. These include its retrospective nature and small sample size. Also, using a method is based on only a part of and not the entire of HBV genome [4].

Restriction fragment mass polymorphism (RFMP) is another method for detecting genotypes. Lee et al. utilized RFMP for HBV genotyping based on genotypic variations in the S gene, which is similar to RFLP. This method depends on restriction enzyme digestion of PCR products to produce genotype specific oligonucleotide fragments. The mass of the produced fragments is then determined using matrix-assisted laser desorption/ionization–time-of-flight (MALDI-TOF) mass spectrometry. Other studies have reported the use of MALDI-TOF mass spectrometry for determination of YMDD (tyrosine–methionine–aspartate–aspartate–motif) mutations, which are linked to lamivudine (LAM) drug resistance [54].

Author details

Ali Adel Dawood
Department of Anatomy, College of Medicine, University of Mosul, Mosul, Iraq

*Address all correspondence to: aad@uomosul.edu.iq

References

[1] Regev A, Schiff ER. Viral hepatitis A. B and C. *Clin Liver Dis*. 2000;**4**:47-71

[2] Tat FS. Development of molecular diagnostic system for detection of hepatitis B virus in blood donations. M.Sc. thesis in Medical Science: University of Hong Kong; 2003

[3] King, AM., Adem, MJ. Carstens, EB and Lefkowitz, EJ. (2011). Report of the International Committee on Taxonomy of Viruses. San Diego: Elsevier Academic Press.

[4] Kumar V, Das S, Jameel S. The biology and pathogenesis of hepatitis viruses. Current science. 2010;**98**(3):312-325

[5] Acharya SK, Batra Y. Hepatitis B Virus Genotypes: Clinical Implications. *Medicine Update*. p. 2005:425-429

[6] Alestig E. Geographic and Genetic Diversity of Hepatitis B. University of Gothenburg; 2011

[7] Chen J, Yin J, Tan, x., Zhang, H., Chen, B., Chang, W., Schaefer, S., and Cao, G. Improved multiplex-PCR to identify hepatitis B virus genotypes A–F and subgenotypes B1, B2, C1 and C2. Journal of Clinical virology. 2007;**38**:238-243

[8] Dienstag, J. (2006). Acute Viral Hepatitis. In: Harrison's principle of internal medicine. Kasper D.L., Braunwald E., Fauci A.S., *et al*. eds. 16th ed., McGraw-Hill. Chapter 37: p: 349-377.

[9] Hou J, Liu Z, Gu F. Epidemiology and Prevention of Hepatitis B Virus Infection. International Journal of medical Science. 2005;**2**(1):50-57

[10] Center for Disease Control and Prevention. (2008). Epidemiology and Prevention of Vaccine-Preventable Diseases. Atkinson W. Hamborsky J., Mclntyre I., Wolfe, S., eds. 10th ed., Washington DC: Public Health Foundation. p: 211-234.

[11] Bajunaid, H.A. (2013). Genetic Variability of Hepatitis B Virus. Ph.D. thesis in Molecular Virology. School of Molecular Medicine Sciences. University of Nottingham.

[12] Germer, J.J., Qutub, M.O., Manderkan, J.N., Mitchell, S., and Yao, J.D.C. (2006). Quantification of Hepatitis B Virus (HBV) DNA with a TaqMan HBV Analyte-Specific Reagent following Sample Processing with the MagNA Pure LC Instrument. *Journal of Clinical Microbiology.* P. 1490-1494.

[13] Franciscus, A. (2008). A Guide to Hepatitis B. www.hbvadvocate.org.

[14] Ganem D, Prince AM. Hepatitis B virus infection-natural history and clinical consequences. N Engl J Med. 2004;**350**:1118-1129

[15] Papatheodoridis G, Buti M, Corenberg M, Janssen H, Mutimer D, Raimando GR. EASL Clinical Practice Guidelines: Management of Chronic hepatitis B virus infection. *Journal of Hepatology.* Vol. 2012;**57**:167-185

[16] Willacy, H. (2013). Hepatitis B. *Patient. Co.Uk.* p. 1-7.

[17] McMahon, B.J. (2004). The Natural History of Chronic Hepatitis B Virus Infection. *Seminar in Liver Disease.* Vol. 24, supplement 1, p. 17-21.

[18] Dickens, C. (2011). Occult Hepatitis B Virus (HBV) Infection in The Chacma Baboon. Ph.D. thesis, Faculty of Health Science, University of the Witwatersrand.

[19] Chan CHY, Tse C-H, Mo F, Koh J, Wong V, Wong G, et al. High Viral Load

and Hepatitis B Virus Subgenotype Ce Are Associated With Increased Risk of Hepatocellular Carcinoma. Journal of Clinical Oncology. 2008;**26**:177-182

[20] Liaw YF. HBeAg seroconversion as an important end point in the treatment of chronic hepatitis B. Hepatol Int. 2009;**3**:425-433

[21] Pujol FH, Navas MCH, P., and Chemin, I. Worldwide genetic diversity of HBV genotypes and risk of hepatocellular carcinoma. CancerLetters. 2009;**286**:80-88

[22] Zuckerman, A.J. (1996). "Hepatitis Viruses". In Baron S, et al. Baron's Medical Microbiology (4th Ed.).University of Texas Medical Branch.ISBN0-9631172-1-1.

[23] Kay A, Zoulim F. Hepatitis B virus genetic variability and evolution. Virus Research. 2007;**127**(2):164-176

[24] Sugauchi F, Mizokami M, Orito E, Ohno T, Kato H, Suzuki S, et al. A novel variant genotype C of hepatitis B virus identified in isolates from Australian Aborigines: complete genome sequence and phylogenetic relatedness. Journal of General Virology. 2001;**82**:883-892

[25] McMahon BJ. The influence of hepatitis B virus genotype and subgenotype. On the natural history of chronic hepatitis B. *Hepatol Int.* 2009;**3**:334-342

[26] Mizokami M, Nakano T, Orito E, Tanaka Y, Sakugawa H, Mukaide M, et al. Hepatitis B virus genotype assignment using restriction fragment length polymorphism patterns. FEBS Letters. 1999;**450**:66-71

[27] Seid KYS. Serological and Molecular Characterization of Hepatitis B, C and D Viruses Infections among Health Professionals in Ras Desta and Tikur Anbessa Hospitals, Addis Ababa, Ethiopia. M.Sc thesis Medical Microbiology. Department of Medical Microbiology: Addis Ababa University; 2006

[28] Wang, Z., Tanaka, Y., Huang, Y., kurbanov, F., Chen, J., Zeng, G., Zhou, B., Mizokami, M., and Hou, J. (2007). Clinical and Virological Characteristics of Hepatitis B Virus Subgenotypes Ba, C1, and C2 in China. *Journal of Clinical Microbiology.* P. 1491-1496.

[29] Sharifi Z, Yari F, Gharebaghiyan A. Sequence Analysis of the Polymerase Gene in Hepatitis B Virus Infected Blood Donors in Iran. Arch Iran Med. 2012;**15**(2):88-90

[30] Stuyver L, Gendt SD, Geyt CV, Zoulim F, Fried M, Schinazi R, et al. A new genotype of hepatitis B virus: complete genome and phylogenetic relatedness. Journal of General virology. 2000;**81**

[31] Moriya, T., Kuramoto, I.S., Yoshizawa, H., and Holland, P.V. (2002). Distribution of Hepatitis B Virus Genotypes among American Blood Donors Determined with a PreS2 Epitope Enzyme-Linked Immunosorbent Assay Kit. *Journal of Clinical Microbiology.* p. 877-880.

[32] Ghosh S, Banerjee P, Deny P, Mondal K, Nandi M, RoyChoudhury A, et al. New HBV subgenotype D9, a novel D/C recombinant, identified in patients with chronic HBeAg-negative infection in Eastern India. Journal of Viral Hepatitis. 2012. DOI: 10.1111/j.1365.2893

[33] Kao JH. Molecular epidemiology of Hepatitis B Virus. Korean J. Intern. Med. 2011;**26**:255-261

[34] Miyakawa Y, Mizokami M. Classifying Hepatitis B Virus Genotypes. Intervirology. 2003;**46**:329-338

[35] Huy, T.T.T., Ngoc, T.T., and Abe, K. (2008). New Complex Recombinant

Genotype of Hepatitis B Virus Identified in Vietnam. *Journal of virology.* P. 5657-5663.

[36] Kurbanov F, Tanaka Y, Kramvis A. When Should "I" Consider a New Hepatitis B Virus Genotype? Journal of Virology. 2008;**82**(16):8241-8242

[37] Xu G, Wei C, Guo Y, Zhang C, Zhang N, Wang G. An analysis of the molecular evolution of Hepatitis B viral genotypes A/B/D using a Bayesian evolutionary method. Virology Journal. 2013;**10**:256

[38] Zekri A-RN, Hafez MM, Mohamed NI, Hassan ZK, El-Sayed MH, Khaled MM, et al. Hepatitis B virus (HBV) genotypes in Egyptian pediatric cancer patients with acute and chronic active HBV infection. Virology Journal. 2007. DOI: 10.1186/1743-422x-4-74

[39] VanHemert, FJ, Zaaijer HL, Berkhout B, and Lukashov VV. (2008). Occult hepatitis B infection: an evolutionary scenario. *Virology J.* 11; 5:146.

[40] Zhao, Y., Zhang, X-Y., Guo, J-J., Zeng, A-Z., Hu, J-L., Huang,. W-X., Shan, Y-L., and Huang, A-L. (2010). Simultaneous Genotyping and Quantification of Hepatitis B Virus for Genotypes B and C by Real-Time PCR Assay. *Journal of Clinical Microbiology.* p. 3690-3697.

[41] Horvat RT. Diagnostic and Clinical Relevance of HBV Mutations. Lab. Medicine. 2010;**42**(8):488-496

[42] Norder H, Courouce AM, Coursaget P, Echevarria JM, Lee SD, Mushahwar IK, et al. Genetic Diversity of Hepatitis B Virus Strains Derived Worldwide: Genotypes, Subgenotypes, and HBsAg Subtypes. Inter. virology. 2004;**47**:289-309

[43] Lusida, M.I., Nugrahaputra, V.E., Soetjipto, Handajani, R., Fujii, M.N., Sasayama, M., Utsumi, T., and Hota, H. (2008). Novel Subgenotypes of Hepatitis B Virus Genotypes C and D in Papua, Indonesia. *Journal of Clinical Microbiology.* P. 2160-2166.

[44] Sakamoto T, Tanaka Y, Orito E, Co J, Clavio J, Sugauchi F, et al. Novel subtypes (subgenotypes) of hepatitis B virus genotypes B and C among chronic liver disease patients in the Philippines. Journal of General Virology. 2006;**87**:1873-1882

[45] Chu, C-J., and Lok, A.S.F. (2002). Clinical Significant of Hepatitis B Virus Genotypes. Hepatology Journal. vol. 35.No. 5, p. 1274-1276.

[46] Hussain M, Chu C, Sablon E, Lok ASF. Rapid and Sensitive Assays for Determination of Hepatitis B Virus (HBV) Genotypes and Detection of HBV Precore and Core Promoter Variants. *Journal of clinical Microbiology.* p. 2003:3699-3705

[47] Haryanto A, Mulyani NS, Widoewati T, Wijayanti N, Hadi P. Molecular genotyping of HBV by using Nested PCR-RFLP among Hepatitis B Patients in Daerah Istimewa Yogyakarta province and surrounding area. International Journal of Biotechnology. 2008;**13**(2):1098-1104

[48] Okamoto H, Tsuda F, Sakugawa H, Sastrosoewignjo RI, Imai M, Miyakawa Y, et al. Typing Hepatitis B Virus by Homology in Nucleotide Sequence: Comparison of Surface Antigen Subtypes. Journal of General Virology. 1988;**69**:2575-2583

[49] Ohnuma, H., Machida, A., Okamoto, H., Tsuda, F., Sakamoto, M., Tanaka, T., Miyakawa, Y., and Mayumi, M. (1993). Allelic Subtypic Determinants of Hepatitis B Surface Antigen (i and t) That Are Distinct from d/y or w/r. *Journal of Virology.* P. 927-932.

[50] Zhang P, Yu M-YW, Venable R, Alter HJ, Shih JW-K. Neutralization epitope responsible for the hepatitis B virus subtype- specific protection in chimpanzees. PNAS. 2006;**103**(24):9214-9219

[51] Cui C, Shi J, Hui L, Xi H, Quni Z, Hu G. The dominant hepatitis B virus genotype identified in Tibet is a C/D hybrid. Journal of General Virology. 2002;**83**:2773-2777

[52] Repp R, Rhiel S, Heermann KH, Schaefer S, Keller C, Ndumbe P, et al. Genotyping By Multiplex Polymerase Chain Reaction for Detection of Endemic hepatitis B Virus Transmission. *Journal of Clinical Microbiology.* p. 1993:1095-1102

[53] Valsamakis A. Molecular Testing in the Diagnosis and Management of Chronic Hepatitis B. Clinical Microbiology Reviews. 2007;**20**:426-439

[54] Guirgis, B.S.S., Abbas, R.O., and Azzazy, H.M.E. (2010). Hepatitis B virus genotyping: current methods and clinical implications. *International Journal of Infectious Diseases.* P: e941-e953.

[55] Osiowy C, Giles E. Evaluation of the INNO-LiPA HBV Genotyping Assay for Determination of Hepatitis B Virus Genotype. *Journal of Clinical Microbiology.* p. 2003:5473-5477

[56] Cabezas Fernandez, M.T., and Cabeza Barrera, M.I. (2012). Introduction of an Automated System for the Diagnosis and Quantification of Hepatitis B and Hepatitis C Viruses. *The Open Virology Journal.* 6, (Suppl 1: M4) p. 122-134.

[57] Ouneissa, R., Bahri, O., Yahia, A.B., Touzi, H., Azouz, M.M., Mami, N. B., and Triki, H. (2013). Evaluation of PCR-RFLP in the Pre-S Region as Molecular Method for Hepatitis B Virus Genotyping. *Hepatitis Monthly.* 13(10):e11781. p. 67-74.

[58] Pas SD, Tran N, de-Man, R.A., Burghoorn-Mass, C., Vernet, G., and Niesters, H.G.M. Comparison of Reverse Hybridization, Microarray, and Sequence Analysis for Genotyping Hepatitis B Virus. *Journal of Clinical Microbiology.* p. 2008:1268-1273

[59] Becker CE, Kretzmann NA, Mattos AA, Veiga ABGD. Screening of Hepatitis B Virus Genotypes A, D and F in Patients from a General Hospital in Southern Brazil. Arq Gastroenterol. 2013;**50**(3):219-225

[60] Tatematsu, K., Tanaka, Y., Kurbanov, F., Sugauchi, F., Mano, S., Maeshiro, T., Nakayoshi, T., wakuta, M., Miyakawa, Y., and Mizokami, M. (2009). A Genetic Variant of Hepatitis B Virus Divergent from Known Human and Ape Genotypes Isolated from a Japanese Patient and Provisionally Assigned to New Genotype J. *Journal of Virology.* P. 10538-10547.

[61] Scheiblauer H, El-Nageh M, Dias S, Nick S, Zeichhardt H, Grunert H, et al. Performance evaluation of 70 hepatitis B virus (HBV) surface antigen (HBsAg) assays from around the world by a geographically diverse panel with an array of HBV genotypes and HBsAg subtypes. The International Journal of Transfusion Medicine. 2009;**98**:403-414

[62] Ciotti M, Marcuccilli F, Guenci T, Prignano MG, Federico C. Evaluation of the Abbott RealTime HBV DNA Assay and Comparison to the Cobas AmpliPrep/Cobas TaqMan 48 Assay in Monitoring Patients with Chronic Cases of Hepatitis B. *Journal of Clinical Microbiology.* p. 2008:1517-1519

[63] Malmstrom S, Berglin-Enquist I, Lindh M. Novel Method for Genotyping Hepatitis B Virus on the Basis of TaqMan Real-Time PCR. *Journal of Clinical Microbiology.* p. 2010:1105-1111

[64] Vargis EA. Virus Detection with DNA logic Tags. M.Sc. thesis in

Biomedical Engineering. Faculty of the Graduate School of Vanderbilt University; 2007

[65] Naito, H., Hayashi, S., and Abe, K. (2001). Rapid and Specific Genotyping System for Hepatitis B Virus Corresponding to Six Major Genotypes by PCR Using Type-Specific Primers. *Journal of Clinical Microbiology*. P. 362-364.

[66] Utsumi T, Lusida MI, Yano Y, Nugrahaputra VE, Amin M, Juniastuti S, et al. Complete Genome Sequence and Phylogenetic Relatedness of Hepatitis B Virus Isolates in Papua. Indonesia. *Journal of clinical Microbiology.* p. 2009:1842-1847

[67] Tanaka, Y., Orito, E., Yuen, MF. Mukaide, M., Sugauchi, F., Ito, K., Ozasa, A., Sakamoto, T., Kurbanov, F., Lai, CL., and Mizokami, M. (2005). Two subtypes (subgenotypes) of hepatitis B virus genotype C: A novel subtyping assay based on restriction fragment length polymorphism. *Hepatology Research.* Doi: 10.1016. p. 1-9.

[68] Vivekanandan, P., Abraham, P., Sridharan, G., Chandy, G., Daniel, D., Raghuraman, S., Daniel, H.D., and Subramaniam, T. (2004). Distribution of Hepatitis B Virus Genotypes in Blood Donors and Chronically Infected Patients in a Tertiary Care Hospital in Southern India.

[69] Hanachi N, Fredj NB, Bahri O, Thibault V, ferjani, A., Gharbi, J., Triki, H., and Boukadido, J. Molecular analysis of HBV genotypes and subgenotypes in the Central-East region of Tunisia. Virology Journal. 2010;7:302

[70] Kaklikkaya, N., Sancaktar, M., Guner, R., Buruk, C.K., Koksal, I., Tosun, I., and Aydin, F. (2012). Hepatitis B virus genotypes and subgenotypes in the Eastern Black Sea region of Turkey. *Saudi Med. Journal.* Vol. 33(6). P. 622-626.

Section 2

Mouse Model of Chronic Hepatitis B

Chapter 3

Establishment of a Mouse Model of Chronic Hepatitis B Virus Infection and Purification of Hepatic Parenchymal and Non-Parenchymal Cells

Yan Yan and Chantsalmaa Davgadorj

Abstract

The use of replication-competent hepatitis B virus (HBV) DNA to construct a mouse model will help explore antiviral treatment strategies for more than 240 million patients infected with HBV worldwide. Eradication of chronic HBV infection can effectively block the adverse consequences of HBV-induced hepatic cirrhosis, failure and carcinoma. The core reason that HBV is difficult to eradicate is that most of infected people develop chronic HBV infection due to the establishment of immune tolerance. Here, we introduce a mouse model of adeno-associated virus (AAV)-HBV transfection, which produces HBV surface antigen (HBsAg) that can be maintained for more than 6 months. During virus replication, intermediates, transcripts, and proteins can be detected in peripheral blood. At the same time, the prerequisite for studying liver disease formation and immunotherapy through *in vitro* experiments is to isolate hepatic subgroup cells. Here, we describe a cell sorting method based on liberase perfusion technology combined with low-speed centrifugation and magnetic bead antibody labeling to purify hepatic parenchymal cells (PCs) and non-parenchymal cells (NPCs) step by step from murine liver, such as hepatic sinusoidal endothelial cells (LSECs) and Kupffer cells (KCs), which will help accelerate the study of the genetic and clearance mechanistic of chronic HBV infection.

Keywords: hepatitis B virus, $CD8^+$ T cell, hepatic parenchymal cell (HPC), hepatic sinusoidal endothelial cell (LSEC), Kupffer cell (KC)

1. Introduction

Hepatitis B virus (HBV) has an extremely narrow host-range, such as humans [1], chimpanzees [2], Mauritian cynomolgus monkey [3], treeshrew [4, 5] and woodchuck [6, 7]. These model thereby can be exploited to investigate viral-host interaction and pathogenesis including acute hepatitis, chronic hepatitis, hepatic fibrosis, hepatic cirrhosis and hepatic carcinoma. There are certain limitations using of these models, due to expensive facilities required, difficult to care and ethics restriction, and the shortage of reagents for measuring host factors and for investigating host immunopathogenesis, such as chimpanzees. Mouse is considered to be a less expensive alternative animal model, but its liver lacks the sodium taurocholate cotransporting polypeptide (NTCP) needed for HBV infection. Although human-NTCP (huNTCP) transgenic mice are considered to be able to construct HBV-infected mice, the results failed to support the original hypothesis by measuring HBV DNA [8].

Studies on the HBV mouse models have gone through several generations, involved in HBV DNA transgenic mice [9], HBV DNA transfected mice [10], HBV rc-cccDNA transfected mice [11], HBV-infected liver chimeric humanized mice and CRISPR/Cas9 technological NRG/Fah−/− immune deficient mice [12]. Their advantages and disadvantages are as follows, separately: (1) 1.3-fold HBV genome transgenic mice support the expression of viral RNA and viral proteins in the liver, and can develop complete pgRNA, viral assembly and viral secretion during in the viral cycle, and support endosomal antiviral [13]. Due to the integration of the HBV genome in the host chromosome, the disadvantages of transgenic mice include the undetectable HBV cccDNA in mouse hepatocytes, the innate immune tolerance to HBV antigens (Ags), and the inability to study Ag-related immune activation. (2) The 1.2-fold HBV genomic DNA hydrodynamic injection (H.I.) model is one major breakthrough and first developed to meet the requirements of mouse nonintegrated viral genomes [14]. Different from immunodeficient mice such as liver humanized mice, the mice can express HBV Ags, and the immune system can also recognize the Ags to stimulate virus-specific immune responses. This model system can be used to test HBV cure strategies and study HBV immunology [15, 16]. However, this mode has limitation of mouse category. For example, experiments have shown that male C3H and C57BL/6 J are more effective, and the success rate varies in mouse models [17, 18]. The operation of H.I. also requires a high level of technical proficiency. The AAV-HBV vector has minimal AAV genome, only the essential AAV inverted terminal repeat sequence (ITR), is used to analyze the virus packaging and does not encode any AAV viral proteins. Therefore, this vector provides a clean background when analyzing HBV-specific immune responses. In our chapter, we will introduce how to establish this mouse model, the detectable HBsAg protein persists in blood or liver more than 6 months and has been widely used as chronic infection model [19]. (3) HBV replication is not detectable and HBV cccDNA non-formation is suggested to be restricted in mouse model [20]. HBV cccDNA is a symbol of continuous virus replication and an indispensable component for HBV to cause liver damage and fibrosis [21]. The half-life of HBV cccDNA is long in the human liver, which is a difficult problem for clinical cure of hepatitis B. Construct a transfected recombinant minicircle cccDNA achieving long-term maintenance in C3H mouse modle contributes to investigating HBV cccDNA-related biology and for evaluating anti-HBV drugs [11]. In order to overcome the shortcoming of cccDNA lasting only a few weeks, a mouse model was constructed using adenovirus vectors and the linear HBV cccDNA genome was delivered to Cre transgenic mouse [22]. (4) Humanized immunodeficient mice have been used to generate HBV-infected mice [23]. However, these animals lace a functional immune system, hindering research on immunological issues related to HBV infection and immunotherapy.

At present, AAV-HBV plasmid transfection can obtain an ideal HBV chronic infection mouse model, and it has been applied in a number of studies [14, 24, 25]. In the clinical recovery process of chronic hepatitis B, there are strict rules on the selectivity of anti-viral therapy for patients to ensure that interferon combined with nucleoside analog therapy produces better results. Therefore, it is necessary to further understand the relationship between drugs, HBV and hepatocyte immunity. As our previous studies have shown, TLRs [26, 27] and chemokines [15, 25] can promote the clearance of HBV by regulating the status of hepatic parenchymal cells (PCs) and non-parenchymal cells (NPCs), and also clarifies the cellular mechanism. Hepatic PCs and NPCs play a key role in mediating liver immune tolerance and mediating early innate and adaptive immune responses. Small molecule drugs or cytokines activate these cells to promote virus clearance. The specific mechanism will be verified using isolated mouse hepatocytes and the corresponding mechanism will be explained.

2. Materials

2.1 Materials for transformation and extraction of plasmids

1. Plasmid: The plasmid pAAV/HBV1.2 (ampicillin resistance) was kindly provided by Prof. Chen Pei-Jer (Graduate Institute of Clinical Medicine, College of Medicine, National Taiwan University, Taiwan), containing 1.2 times of the full-length DNA HBV genome [28].

2. Sterilized 100 mL liquid Luria Broth (LB) bacterial medium and 50 mL Luria Agar (LA) (1.5–2% agar, 0.75–1 g) solid bacterial medium [29]. LB medium: Tryptone 1 g/L, Yeast extract 0.5 g/L, NaCl 1 g/L, pH 7.4. The final volume of the solution is up to 100 mL.

3. 50 μL competent *E.coli* DH5α strain bath in broken ice (Laboratory preparation or purchase).

4. Sterilized ddH_2O, 1 mol/L $CaCl_2$, 0.6 mol/L $MgCl_2$ and sterile 50 μg/mL ampicillin (Amp) (Invitrogen).

5. Water bath at 42°C.

6. A horizontal shaker with constant temperature at 37°C.

7. 5% CO_2, 37°C incubator for bacterial culture.

8. NucleoBond Xtra Maxi EF, Maxi kit for endotoxin-free plasmid DNA kits (Macherey-Nagel).

9. 4% paraformaldehyde: 4 g paraformaldehyde powder is dissolved in PBS at 56°C, stored at room temperature and protected from light.

2.2 Materials, reagents and culture media for hepatocyte extraction and culture

1. Mice: 6–8 weeks old male C57BL/6 J are bred and maintained under specific pathogen-free (SPF) conditions in the Animal Research Center.

2. Water bath at 37°C.

3. Sterile 50 mL conical centrifuge tubes, 25 mL disposable plastic pipettes and adjustable pipette device.

4. Disposable 70 μm filters or reusable stainless steel meshes.

5. Sterile 10-cm bacteria or cell petri dishes.

6. A 50 mL beaker containing surgical instruments soaked in 75% alcohol, several pairs of ophthalmological scissors and fine-pointed ophthalmological tweezers.

Perfusion buffer and medium	Reagent ingredient	Total amount	Proportion
Liberase digestive medium (LDM)	Liberase powder	50 mg	−20°C
	GBSS buffer	7.14 mL	300 μL/tube (aliquot)
Liver perfusion medium (LPM)	LDM	300 μL/ tube	−20°C
	GBSS buffer	30 mL	
Liver cell digestion medium (LCDM)	DMEM (High glucose)	500 mL	
	Hepes (1 mol/L)	7.5 mL	15 mmol/L
	Penicillin (100 ×)	5 mL	1%
Hepatocyte culture medium (HCM)	Williams' Medium	500 mL	Sigma-Aldrich
	Fetal bovine serum	50 mL	10%
	100 × L-glutamine (Glu)	5 mL	1%
	Hepes (1 mol/L)	2.5 mL	5 mmol/L
	Penicillin (100 ×)	5 mL	1%
	DMSO	10 mL	2%
	Hydrocortisone		0.05 nM
	Insulin		5 μL/mL
	100 × None essential amino acid (NEAA)	5 mL	1%
LSEC/KC medium	DMEM (High glucose)	500 mL	
	Fetal bovine serum	50 mL	10%
	100 × L-Glu (glutamine)	5 mL	1%
	Hepes (1 mol/L)	2.5 mL	5 mmol/L

Table 1.
Formulas of perfusion and hepatocyte culture media.

7. 75% ethanol, adjustable-speed peristaltic pump and perfusion connection line device (27 gauge 1.25 inch needles).

8. 24-well and 48-well culture plates pre-coated with mouse collagenase type II (Sigma-Aldrich), rinse 3–4 times with PBS before use.[1]

9. Sterilized 1 L phosphate buffered saline (PBS, calcium- and magnesium-free): 7.9 g NaCl, 0.2 g KCl, 0.24 g Na_2HPO_4 and 1.8 g K_2HPO_4, pH 7.4.

[1] Dilute 5 mg rat tail collagen type II with 1 mL 0.006 mol/L (0.36 g/L) sterile acetic acid solution, and dissolve 240 μL of collagen II (5 mg /mL) to 95 mL sterile acetic acid solution, and finally dilute to 100 mL. Dissolve the rat tail collagen type II solution used for coating at 5–8 $\mu g/cm^2$ (cm^2 refers to the bottom surface area of the culture well) (12 μg/mL). Add 300 μL to each well of 24 well plate, and add 150 μL to each well of 48 well plate, then dry overnight under ultraviolet light. The dried plates are kept sealed and can be stored stably for several months (>3 months) at 4–25°C.

10. Sterilized Gey's balanced salt solution (GBSS, calcium-free): 0.14 mM NaCl, 5 mM KCl, 0.3 mM $MgSO_4$, 1 mM Na_2HPO_4, 3 mM $NaHCO_3$, 0.2 mM KH_2PO_4, 1 mM $MgCl_2$, 5.5 mM glucose, pH 7.4.

11. The formulas of digestive enzymes, culture media and drugs are shown in **Table 1**.

12. 0.2% trypan blue, a hemacytometer, a cover glass and a large amount of absorbent tissues.

13. MACS buffer: 1 × PBS adds a total volume of 0.05% bovine serum albumin (BSA) and 2 ml EDTA·Na_2 (0.5 M), pH 7.2.

14. PE rat anti-mouse CD146 antibody (Ab), biotin anti-mouse-F4/80 Ab, anti-PE magnetic beads and streptavidin magnetic beads.

15. BD IMag™ Cell Separation Magnet (BD Biosciences) or MACS separator plus LS Columns (Miltenyi Biotec).

16. 5% CO_2, 37°C incubator for cell culture.

17. Optional: Pentobarbital.

3. Method

3.1 Plasmid enlargement culture and extraction from bacteria

1. 2 μL pAAV/HBV1.2 mix with 45 μL ddH2O, 2.5 μL $CaCl_2$ (1 mol/L), 2.5 μL $MgCl_2$ (0.6 mol/L), then added 50 μL competent *E.coli* DH5α strain, and bathe in ice. Transformation conditions: ice bath 40 min, 42°C heat shock 1.5 min, ice bath 2 min. Add 0.8 mL LB medium, shake for 1 h at 37°C, then centrifugation at 6000 r/min for 5 min, discard the supernatant and inoculate 200 μL transformation bacteria on LB solid medium (Amp^+), and incubate approximate 16 h at 37°C.

2. The target plasmids are extracted as directed by the Macherey-Nagel manufacturer's instructions. The user manual can be downloaded from the website: https://www.mn-net.com/nucleobond-xtra-maxi-kit-for-transfection-grade-plasmid-dna-740414.50?c=3889. Plasmid DNA is divided and stored below −20°C. Detection of DNA concentration before use.[2]

3.2 Mouse model

1. 10 μg of pAAV/HBV1.2 plasmid are injected (H.I.) into the mouse tail veins in a volume of PBS equivalent to 10% of their body weights (g) (v/w) is completed within 5 s [10, 30].

2. HBV replication in the injected mouse serum: Blood specimens are taken from the cheeks of H.I. mice and used to detect hepatitis B surface antigens (HBsAg), hepatitis B e antigens (HBeAg), hepatitis B surface antibodies (anti-HBs), or hepatitis B core antibodies (anti-HBs) at 2 weeks post injection [10].

---

[2] Send the diluted 20 μL DNA for sequencing or real-time PCR to verify accuracy.

Serum levels of HBsAg, HBeAg and HBsAb are detected with ELISA according to the reagent instructions (Jingmei Biotechnology).

3. HBV transcription in the liver: The mouse liver is used to preserve in 4% polyformaldehyde for the next immunohistochemical analysis [10, 25] (Another alternative detection method.[3]

3.3 Perfusion and digestion of mouse liver

1. Biosecurity cabinet and perfusion labs for pre-ultraviolet disinfection.

2. Warm up the PBS and LPM at 37°C, at least 15 mL per mouse per reagent.

3. Install the needle at one end of the perimeter pump line, rinse the line with 75% ethanol for 20 min, then rinse with PBS to remove residual ethanol.

4. Prepare a 10 cm sterile petri dish containing 10 mL of LCDM for liver cell separation and cleaning in the biosecurity cabinet, and an ice box to place cell samples from liver separation on ice. The spare LCDM is also placed in the ice box.

5. Anesthetize or kill the mouse. In the reclining position, according to the previous description [31], the limbs of the mouse are secured with tape on the foam work platform and operated under sterile conditions.[4]

6. Clean the outer surface of the mouse's chest and abdomen with alcohol. The whole process is fast and leaves no blank spots. The skin is the main source of contamination. Use surgical instruments to cut the mouse's abdominal fur in a semicircle below shape, turn it upside down and secure the peritoneum with a surgical instrument.

7. Find the inlet vein of the liver, check the pipes for bubbles, insert a fine needle from the distal end of the inlet vein, and secure the position of the needle. Perfuse the liver tissue with PBS at a speed of 3-5 mL/min, and then cut off the inferior cavity vein after a few seconds. After removing the thrombosis and completing the complete PBS perfusion and 15 mL LPM continuous perfusion.[5,6,7]

---

[3] Detect the level of nucleocapsid HBV DNA extracted from 60 mg of murine liver by real-time PCR on the ABI PRISM 7500 Sequence Detection System (ABI PRISM™). Use an All-In-One DNA/RNA/Protein Mini-preps kit (Sangon Biotech) to purify total DNA from serum. According to the manufacturer's instructions, use careHBV PCR Assay V3 reagents (QIAGEN, China) for HBV DNA detection. This type of model chronic HBV mice has no liver damage and abnormal serum alanine aminotransferase (ALT).

[4] Using tape instead of puncture fixation can reduce the pain of mice and also prevent the mice from waking up from anesthesia as soon as possible.

[5] Before starting priming, carefully check and remove any visible air bubbles in the pump system. Properly activating the pump and piercing the needle into the portal vein to remove any invisible air in the needle tip area may block the microcapillaries and cause insufficient perfusion of certain liver lobes.

[6] This is a non-circulatory perfusion, and all liquid will flow out of the inferior vena cava. Therefore, it is necessary to lay some absorbent tissues on the foam workbench where the mouse is fixed.

[7] Perfusion and digestion are very important steps. During the digestion process, digestive enzymes are injected and the severed inferior vena cava is pressed to close the vascular output, so that the liver is fully perfused and expanded, which can prolong the effective digestion time. After ideal digestion, the liver will turn from red to yellow-white, and the tissues will become soft after digestion. The more complete the liver digestion, the higher the ratio of single cells to live hepatic parenchymal cells, and the higher the survival rate in culture.

8. After perfusion, clamp the digested liver tissue with ophthalmic tweezer, cut off the connective tissue around it with slight operation, and place it in the dish containing LCDM in biosecurity cabinet.

9. Firstly, peel off the gallbladder. Using two sets of disinfection ophthalmic tweezers to gently scrape the liver capsule, gently shake the liver tissue to release the digested single cells, and 10 mL LCDM becomes muddy, only a small amount of fibrous tissue remaining is the ideal digestion process.[8]

3.4 Isolation and culture of hepatocytes

1. Transfer the hepatocyte suspension to a new 50 mL centrifuge tube via a 70 μm filter. Wash the 10 cm petri dish 2–3 times with 15 mL LCDM and transfer to the 50 mL conical centrifuge tube via the same 70 μm filter.

2. **Hepatic PCs:** After isolating all mouse hepatocytes, the hepatocyte suspension can be placed on ice.

    i. Spin the cells at 50 g at 4°C for 5 min, 3 times, and wash with hepatocyte culture medium (HCM); Centrifuge has 9 speeds of acceleration and 9 speeds of decelerates (i.e., acceleration of 9, deceleration of 9).

    ii. Aspirate the supernatant into a new 50 mL centrifuge tube. The supernatant contains hepatic non-parenchymal cells (NPCs).[9] The precipitated cells are hepatic PCs.

    iii. Inoculate hepatic PCs on a 24-well plates covered with collagen II, 360 μL/well (Use HCM to dilute PCs to 3.5×10^6 cells/ml before inoculation).

    iv. Incubate at 37°C, 5% CO2, and shake at the crossover level every 15 min for 1 h to suspend the hepatocytes with lower viability. Incubate overnight, wash with PBS 3 times, change the medium and continue culturing. The morphology of hepatic PCs is shown in **Figure 1**.[10]

4. Hepatic NPCs (LSECs/KCs)

i. Spin hepatic NPCs at 4°C, 300 g for 10 min; Accelerate by 9, decelerate by 9; Discard the supernatant and gently scrape the bottom to allow the cells to

[8] Do not damage the gallbladder during the entire process of liver separation, as this will reduce the production and viability of hepatic parenchymal cells. After the liver is digested, only a small amount of fibrous tissue remains, which means it is in the best digestion state.

[9] The supernatant of hepatic PCs of the same mouse each time washing may contain target hepatic NPCs, all of which are mixed together for subsequent cell sorting.

[10] Experimental results show that the survival rate of mouse liver parenchymal hepatocytes needs to reach more than 70%, and a better survival rate can be obtained after culture. Mature hepatocytes mostly have two nuclei and three nuclei. In addition, even if washed with PBS, dead cells will still exist.

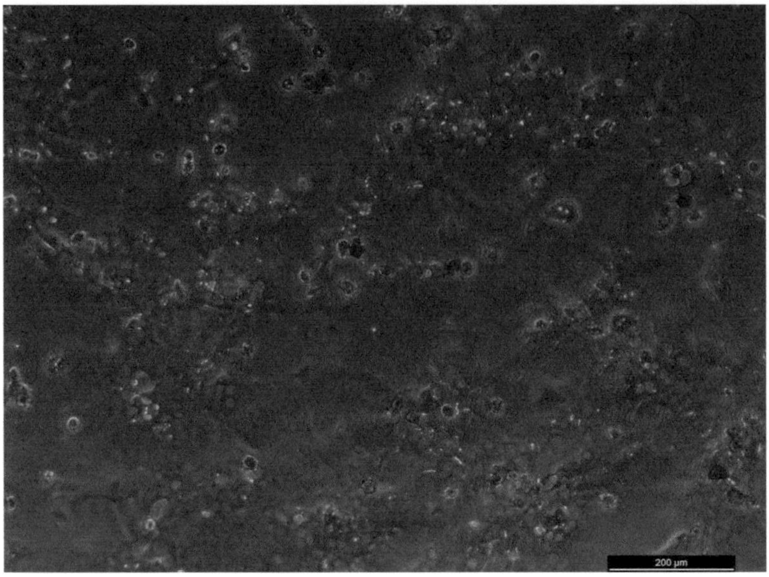

Figure 1.
hepatic PCs cultured for 48 h

suspend; Wash the NPCs with 50 mL MACS buffer, pick out if there are dead cells or tissue clumps, centrifuge as above, discard the supernatant, and gently scrape the bottom.

ii. Add the selected PE rat anti-mouse CD146 Ab solution (2.5 μL Ab +250 mL MACS per liver) to the cell suspension for labeling LSECs, protected from light.

iii. Incubate at 4°C for 20 min or at room temperature for 30 min.

iv. Add more than 10 times the volume of MACS buffer to the incubated cells for washing.

v. Spin NPCs at 4°C，300 g for 10 min; Accelerate by 9, decelerate by 9; Discard the supernatant and gently scrape the bottom to allow the cells to suspend.

vi. Add 20 μL of anti-PE magnetic bead to 180 μL of MACS buffer in each liver specimen.

vii. Incubate at 4°C for 15 min, add 10 times the volume of MACS buffer, and spin at 4°C, 300 g for 10 min.

viii. Discard the supernatant, supplement with MACS until the number of cells is 1–8 × 10^7cells/mL, put it in one or more flow cytometry tubes and immediately place them on the BD IMag™ Cell Separation Magnet for 8–10 min to attract the cells labeled with magnetic beads; keep the flow tubes on the magnetic stand, and carefully aspirate the supernatants to a new 50 mL tube. Using the same suction method, suspend and clean the old tube twice with MACS. The negative cells in the supernatants can be collected in a new tube.

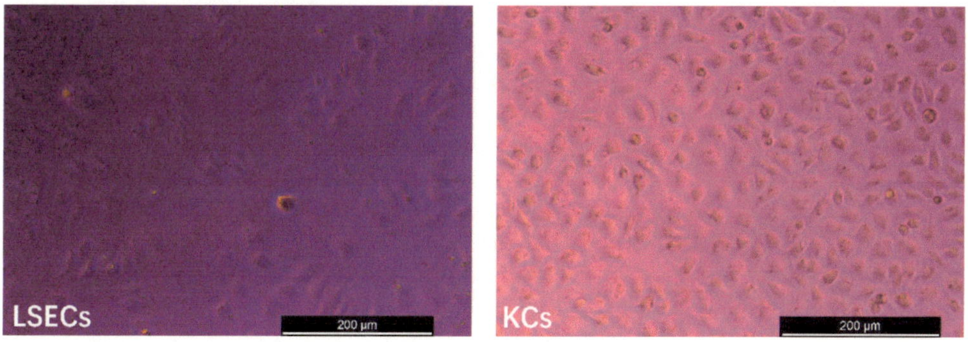

Figure 2.
hepatic NPCs cultured for 48 h.

ix. Add 1 mL LSEC culture medium to suspend the cells. After counting, inoculate the diluted LSECs (1×10^6/mL) into a 48-well plate pre-coated with collagen II, and inoculate 500 µL per well.

x. Spin the liquid collected in step viii with a 50 mL tube at 4°C and 300 g for 10 min, and discard the supernatant. Gently scrape the bottom to suspend the cells and add 2.5 µL biotin anti-mouse-F4/80 Ab MACS solution (2.5 µL Ab +250 mL MACS per liver).

xi. Refer to steps iii-v for antibody incubation and washing, and add 20 µL streptavidin magnetic bead to 180 µL MACS buffer in each liver specimen.

xii. Incubation and magnetic attraction are the same as steps vii-viii to obtain F4/80$^+$ KCs. Add 1 mL KC culture medium to suspend the cells. After counting, inoculate the diluted KCs (1×10^6/mL) into a 96-well plate with 200 µL per well.

xiii. Both LSECs and KCs need to be cultured overnight in a 5% CO_2 37°C incubator. The next day, wash with PBS 3 times, and add DMEM complete medium the next day. The cell morphology of LSECs and KCs is shown in **Figure 2.**[11]

Acknowledgements

We thank Professor Pei-Jer Chen from National Taiwan University for presenting the plasmid pAAV/HBV1.2. This work was supported by the National Natural Science Foundation of China (81701550), the Top Talent Support Program for Young and Middle-Aged People of Wuxi Health Committee (BJ2020094), and the Wuxi Key Medical Talents Program (ZDRC024).

[11] The isolated NPCs can be verified by flow cytometry in a small amount: the cell surface markers of NPCs are stained for flow cytometry analysis as described previously [31]. Briefly, LSEC (CD146$^+$) and KCs (CD45$^-$, IA/IE$^+$, and F4/80$^+$) can be detected by flow cytometry assay. All Abs are purchased from BD biosciences and eBioscience. The flow test results are analyzed using FlowJo 11.0.

Conflict of interest

The authors declare no conflict of interest.

Author details

Yan Yan[1,2*] and Chantsalmaa Davgadorj[1]

1 Laboratory for Infection and Immunity, The Fifth People's Hospital of Wuxi, Affiliated Hospital of Jiangnan University, Wuxi, China

2 Hepatology Institute of Wuxi, The Fifth People's Hospital of Wuxi, Affiliated Hospital of Jiangnan University, Wuxi, China

*Address all correspondence to: yanyan198134@hotmail.com

References

[1] Francis VC. Mint: Hepatitis B virus immunopathogenesis. Annu Rev Immunol. 1995; 13: 29-60. DOI: 10.1146/annurev.iy.13.040195.000333

[2] Guidotti LG, Rochford R, Chung J, Shapiro M, Purcell R, Chisari FV. Mint: Viral clearance without destruction of infected cells during acute HBV infection. Science. 1999; 284: 825-829. DOI: 10.1126/science.284.5415.825

[3] Dupinay T, Gheit T, Roques P, Cova L, Chevallier-Queyron P, Tasahsu SI, Le Grand R, Simon F, Cordier G, Wakrim L, Benjelloun S, Trepo C, Chemin I. Mint: Discovery of naturally occurring transmissible chronic hepatitis B virus infection among Macaca fascicularis from Mauritius Island. Hepatology. 2013; 58: 1610-1620. DOI: 10.1002/hep.26428

[4] Yan R, Su J, Huang D, Gan Y, Yang C, Huang G. Mint: Human hepatitis B virus and hepatocellular carcinoma I. Experimental infection of tree shrews with hepatitis B virus. Journal of Cancer Research and Clinincal Oncology. 1996; 122: 283-288. DOI: 10.1007/BF01261404

[5] Kock J, Nassal M, MacNelly S, Baumert TF, Blum HE, von Weizsacker F. Mint: Efficient infection of primary tupaia hepatocytes with purified human and woolly monkey hepatitis B virus. Journal of Virology. 2001; 75: 5084-5089. DOI: 10.1128/JVI.75.11.5084-5089.2001

[6] Kulkarni K, Jacobson IM, Tennant BC. Mint: The role of the woodchuck model in the treatment of hepatitis B virus infection. Clinics in Liver Disease. 2007; 11: 707-725, vii. DOI: 10.1016/j.cld.2007.08.012

[7] Yan Q, Li M, Liu Q, Li F, Zhu B, Wang J, Lu Y, Liu J, Wu J, Zheng X, Lu M, Wang B, Yang D. Mint: Molecular characterization of woodchuck IFI16 and AIM2 and their expression in woodchucks infected with woodchuck hepatitis virus (WHV). Scientific Reports. 2016; 6: 28776. DOI: 10.1038/srep28776

[8] Li H, Zhuang Q, Wang Y, Zhang T, Zhao J, Zhang Y, Zhang J, Lin Y, Yuan Q, Xia N, Han J. Mint: HBV life cycle is restricted in mouse hepatocytes expressing human NTCP. Cellular & Molocular Immunology. 2014; 11: 175-183. DOI: 10.1038/cmi.2013.66

[9] Chisar FV. Mint: Hepatitis B virus transgenic mice insights into the virus and the disease. Hepatology. 1990; 22: 1316-1325. DOI: 10.1016/0270-9139(95) 90645-2

[10] Huang LR, Wu HL, Chen PJ, Chen DS. Mint: An immunocompetent mouse model for the tolerance of human chronic hepatitis B virus infection. Proceedings of the National Academy of Sciences of the United States of America. 2006; 103: 17862-17867. DOI: 10.1073/pnas.0608578103

[11] Yan Z, Zeng J, Yu Y, Xiang K, Hu H, Zhou X, Gu L, Wang L, Zhao J, Young JAT, Gao L. Mint: HBVcircle: A novel tool to investigate hepatitis B virus covalently closed circular DNA. Journal of Hepatology. 2017; 66: 1149-1157. DOI: 10.1016/j.jhep.2017.02.004

[12] Li F, Cowley DO, Banner D, Holle E, Zhang L, Su L. Mint: Efficient genetic manipulation of the NOD-Rag1-/-IL2RgammaC-null mouse by combining in vitro fertilization and CRISPR/Cas9 technology. Scientific Reports. 2014; 4: 5290. DOI: 10.1038/srep05290

[13] Uprichard SL, Boyd B, Althage A, Chisari FV. Mint: Clearance of hepatitis B virus from the liver of transgenic mice by short hairpin RNAs. Proceedings of the National Academy of Sciences of the

United States of America. 2005; 102: 773-778. DOI: 10.1073/pnas.0409028102

[14] Yang PL, Althage A, Chung J, Chisari FV. Mint: Hydrodynamic injection of viral DNA: a mouse model of acute hepatitis B virus infection. Proceedings of the National Academy of Sciences of the United States of America. 2002; 99: 13825-13830. DOI: 10.1073/pnas.202398599

[15] Liu C, Huang X, Werner M, Broering R, Ge J, Li Y, Liao B, Sun J, Peng J, Lu M, Hou J, Zhang X. Mint: Elevated expression of chemokine CXCL13 in chronic hepatitis B patients links to immune control during antiviral therapy. Frontiers in Immunology. 2017; 8: 323. DOI: 10.3389/fimmu.2017.00323

[16] Freitas AA, Dietze KK, Schimmer S, Kretzmer F, Wang J, Lin Y, Huang X, Wu W, Wang B, Lu M, Dittmer U, Yang D, Liu J. Mint: Characterization of the Treg response in the hepatitis B virus hydrodynamic injection mouse model. Plos One. 2016; 11: e0151717. DOI: 10.1371/journal.pone.0151717

[17] Peng XH, Ren XN, Chen LX, Shi BS, Xu CH, Fang Z, Liu X, Chen JL, Zhang XN, Hu YW, Zhou XH. Mint: High persistence rate of hepatitis B virus in a hydrodynamic injection-based transfection model in C3H/HeN mice. World Journal of Gastroenterology. 2015; 21: 3527-3536. DOI:10.3748/wjg.v21.i12.3527

[18] Yang D, Liu L, Zhu D, Peng H, Su L, Fu YX, Zhang L. Mint: A mouse model for HBV immunotolerance and immunotherapy. Cellular & Molecular Immunology. 2014; 11: 71-78. DOI: 10.1038/cmi.2013.43

[19] Dion S, Bourgine M, Godon O, Levillayer F, Michel ML. Mint: Adeno-associated virus-mediated gene transfer leads to persistent hepatitis B virus replication in mice expressing HLA-A2 and HLA-DR1 molecules. Journal of Virology. 2013; 87: 5554-5563. DOI: 10.1128/JVI.03134-12

[20] Lucifora J, Salvetti A, Marniquet X, Mailly L, Testoni B, Fusil F, Inchauspe A, Michelet M, Michel ML, Levrero M, Cortez P, Baumert TF, Cosset FL, Challier C, Zoulim F, Durantel D. Mint: Detection of the hepatitis B virus (HBV) covalently-closed-circular DNA (cccDNA) in mice transduced with a recombinant AAV-HBV vector. Antiviral Research. 2017; 145: 14-19. DOI: 10.1016/j.antiviral.2017.07.006

[21] Rehermann B, Ferrari C, Pasquinelli C, Chisari FV. Mint: The hepatitis B virus persists for decades after patients' recovery from acute viral hepatitis despite active maintenance of a cytotoxic T-lymphocyte response. Nature Medicine. 1996; 2: 1104–1108. DOI: 10.1038/nm1096-1104

[22] Li G, Zhu Y, Shao D, Chang H, Zhang X, Zhou D, Gao Y, Lan K, Deng Q. Mint: Recombinant covalently closed circular DNA of hepatitis B virus induces long-term viral persistence with chronic hepatitis in a mouse model. Hepatology. 2018; 67: 56-70. DOI: 10.1002/hep.29406

[23] Allweiss L, Dandri M. Mint: Experimental in vitro and in vivo models for the study of human hepatitis B virus infection. Journal of Hepatology. 2016; 64: S17-S31. DOI: 10.1016/j.jhep.2016.02.012

[24] Song J, Li S, Zhou Y, Liu J, Francois S, Lu M, Yang D, Dittmer U, Sutter K. Mint: Different antiviral effects of IFNalpha subtypes in a mouse model of HBV infection. Scientific Reports. 2017; 7: 334. DOI: 10.1038/s41598-017-00469-1

[25] Yan Y, Zhao W, Liu W, Li Y, Wang X, Xun J, Davgadorj C. Mint: CCL19 enhances CD8+ T-cell responses

and accelerates HBV clearance. Journal of Gastroenterology. 2021; 56: 769-785. DOI: 10.1007/s00535-021-01799-8

[26] Ma Z, Cao Q, Xiong Y, Zhang E, Lu M. Mint: Interaction between hepatitis B virus and Toll-like receptors: current status and potential therapeutic use for chronic hepatitis B. Vaccines. 2018; 6: 6. DOI: 10.3390/vaccines6010006

[27] Wu J, Meng Z, Jiang M, Pei R, Trippler M, Broering R, Bucchi A, Sowa J-P, Dittmer U, Yang D, Roggendorf M, Gerken G, Lu M, Schlaak JF. Mint: Hepatitis B virus suppresses toll-like receptor-mediated innate immune responses in murine parenchymal and nonparenchymal liver cells. Hepatology. 2009; 49: 1069-1082. DOI: 10.1002/hep.22773

[28] Lin YJ, Huang LR, Yang HC, Tzeng HT, Hsu PN, Wu HL, Chen PJ, Chen DS. Mint: Hepatitis B virus core antigen determines viral persistence in a C57BL/6 mouse model. Proceedings of the National Academy of Sciences of the United States of America. 2010; 107: 9340-9345. DOI: 10.1073/pnas.1004762107

[29] MacWilliams MP, Liao M-K (2006) Luria broth (LB) and luria agar (LA) media and their uses protocol.

[30] Lin Y, Huang X, Wu J, Liu J, Chen M, Ma Z, Zhang E, Liu Y, Huang S, Li Q, Zhang X, Hou J, Yang D, Lu M, Xu Y. Mint: Pre-activation of Toll-like receptor 2 enhances CD8+ T-cell responses and accelerates hepatitis B virus clearance in the mouse models. Frontiers in Immunology. 2018; 9: 1495. DOI: 10.3389/fimmu.2018.01495

[31] Yan Y, Hu K, Deng X, Guan X, Luo S, Tong L, Du T, Fu M, Zhang M, Liu Y, Hu Q. Mint: Immunization with HSV-2 gB-CCL19 fusion constructs protects mice against lethal vaginal challenge. The Journal of Immunology. 2015; 195: 329-338. DOI: 10.4049/jimmunol.1500198

Section 3

Levels of Antibody Response against HBV

Chapter 4

Level of Antibody Response against Hepatitis B Virus after Vaccination and Seroprevalence of HBV in Children Addis Ababa, Ethiopia

Habtamu Biazin Kebede and Seifegebriel Teshome

Abstract

Approximately 2 billion people worldwide are infected with HBV and more than 240 million are chronic carriers. The World Health Organization officially launched the introduction of the hepatitis B vaccine for children in 1980. Since then, different countries have determined the level of response to the vaccine. Since the introduction of the vaccine in Ethiopia in 2007, there have been few studies evaluating the antibody response to the HBV vaccine. Therefore, the purpose of this study is to determine the HBV antibody response after hepatitis B vaccination and to evaluate the HBV seroprevalence of children in Addis Ababa, Ethiopia. A cross-sectional study was conducted using a multistage probability sampling technique. Four hundred and fifty children between the ages of five and eight living in Addis Ababa were enrolled. Socio-demographic characteristics were obtained through a structured questionnaire and three to four ml of blood was collected from each child. ELISA was performed to determine antibody levels against HBV. The average age is seven + one (SD) years. Anti-HBs were detected in 54.3% (208/450) of children, and girls 98 (54.7%) had a slightly higher level of protection than boys 110 did (53.9%). The overall coverage rate of the vaccine in this study was 85.1%. The proportion of children with protective levels (> 10 mIU / ml of anti-HBs antibodies) decreased with increasing age of the children: 5, 6, 7 and 8 years were 52.6%, 60%, 43.5% and 37.1%, respectively. The seroprevalence rate for HBsAg is 0.4% and the seroprevalence rate for anti-HBc is 5.6%. Age and antibody response level were negatively correlated ($p = 0.001$), while gender and history of HBV infection were not significantly correlated. Age was also significantly correlated with anti-HBc seropositivity ($p = 0.003$). HBV vaccine coverage for children is high, but the antibody response to the vaccine appears to be low. The seropositivity rate for the virus is also very low. Low levels of response to the vaccine should be a problem. For unresponsive children, revaccination or booster doses should be considered. More research needs to be done.

Keywords: HBV, antibody response level, vaccination status, HBsAg, Anti HBsAg, Anti HBc

1. Introduction

Hepatitis B virus (HBV) infection is a serious global health concern. Around two billion people have been infected with HBV worldwide, and more than 257 million people are currently living with hepatitis B virus infection [1]. There are an estimated 600,000 deaths annually from complications of HBV-related liver diseases [2]. The highest numbers of HBsAg carriers are found in developing countries with limited medical facilities. Endemicity levels of chronic HBV infection are classified as high (>8%), intermediate (2-8%), or low (<2%). Based on this classification, sub-Saharan African countries including Ethiopia are considered regions of high endemicity [1].

HBV infection can be prevented by using the HBV vaccine. HBV vaccine has been commercially avail- able since the 1980s. In 1991, WHO recommended the integration of the HBV vaccine into the national immunization programs and by the end of 2005, the vaccine coverage was 82.3% globally [3, 4]. Hepatitis B vaccine for infants had been introduced in 183 countries by the end of 2013. In 2007, almost all sub-Saharan African countries had Hepatitis B vaccination in their national program [5]. HBV vaccine was introduced into the Ethiopian Expanded Program of Immunization (EPI) in 2007 and national coverage had reached 86% by 2015 [6].

Immune response to the vaccine can be determined by measuring the concentration of antibodies against the HBsAg. Anti-HBs in vaccinated children decline with time, especially during the first few years of vaccination. Most children produce a high concentration of antibodies following vaccination; however, few children can have low or no response to the vaccine. The reason for this low or no response against the HBV vaccine is not well known. However, the site of injection and modes of administration are thought to be critical factors in achieving an optimal response [7]. Data on the level of immune responses against HBV vaccine in Ethiopia is very limited. This study was conducted to contribute to the base- line data needed for further monitoring of HBV vaccination effectiveness in Ethiopia and provides information on the level of immune responses against HBV vaccine among children in Addis Ababa.

2. Patients and methods

2.1 Study area and period

The study was conducted in Addis Ababa, which is the capital city of Ethiopia from April 2016 to May 2017. A total number of 450 children (5-8 years old) were recruited.

2.2 Study design

A prospective cross-sectional study design was used. Healthy appearing 5-8 years old children were included in the study following their parents' consent. Vaccination status was used to include and exclude participants.

2.3 Sample size determination and sampling technique

The required samples size for this study was calculated using 50% of prevalence in vaccine response using the following formula:

$$n = \frac{\left(\frac{Z\alpha}{2}\right)^2 pq}{d^2} \tag{1}$$

where, n = sample size
q = 1 − p
p = proportion
Z = confidence interval.
Using confidence interval of 95%, Z = 1.96

$$N = \frac{(1.96)^2 * 0.5 * 0.5}{(0.5)^2} = 385 \quad (2)$$

The total number of the samples with 10% non- respondents should come to 424. However, just to be safe we collected 450 samples.

2.4 Data collection

There was a structured questionnaire to collect all relevant information about the study participants. After the participant's family agreed to take part in the study, they signed an in- formed consent form. 3-4 ml of blood sample was collected from each child and the serum was separated and stored at -20°C until further use.

2.5 Ethical clearance

Ethical clearance was obtained from the AHRI/ALERT Research Ethics Review Committee and the department of ethical research committee. A support letter was obtained from the Addis Ababa Health Bureau and from the health bureaus of each sub city. Written informed consent was obtained from each participant's parent or guardian before enrollment.

2.6 Data analysis and interpretation

SPSS Software statistical package version 20.0 was used to analyze the data. Association was determined by Chi-square test. P-values less than 0.05 were considered as statistically significant.

2.7 Serological assays

Serum level HBsAg, anti-HBc, and anti-HBsAg were determined using sandwich ELISA, where antigens/monoclonal antibodies were used both for capture and detection. All ELISA experiments were performed using BIO-RAD, Monolisa ELISA test kits, France. The test kits have a high sensitivity and specificity and each test procedure was undertaken according to the manufacturer's instruction based on standard operating procedures.

2.8 Operational definitions

Hepatitis B virus*:* A DNA virus that attacks the liver and can cause both acute and chronic disease.

HBsAg*:* It is the surface antigen of the hepatitis B virus. It indicates the presence of active hepatitis B infection.

Anti-HBsAg*:* An antibody that is produced against HBV infection or vaccination.

Anti-HBsAg: An antibody that indicates previous or ongoing infection with the hepatitis B virus in an undefined period.

3. Results

3.1 Socio-demographic characteristics

The mean age of the study participants was 7 ± 1 (SD) years. Among these, 244 (54.2%) were male and 383 (85.1%) had been vaccinated. Forty-nine (10.9%) children had a history of infectious disease, fifteen (3.3%) had a history of noninfectious disease, while three (0.7%) were HIV positive (**Table 1**).

Characteristics	Categories	Number (n)	Percentage
Sex	Male	204	54.2
	Female	206	45.8
Age	5	95	21.1
	6	130	28.9
	7	124	27.6
	8	101	22.4
Place of birth	Urban	422	93.8
	Rural	28	6.2
Sub city	Gulele	45	10
	Kirkos	92	20.4
	Lideta	313	69.5
History of previous disease status	Yes	66	14.7
	No	384	85.3
	Infectious	49	10.9
Disease type	Non Infectious	15	3.3
	Immunocompromised	3	0.7
	None	383	85.1
Vaccination status	Vaccinated for HBV	383	85.1
	Non vaccinated for HBV	67	14.9

Table 1.
Socio demographic characteristics of children between the age of 5 and 8 years old in Addis Ababa Ethiopia.

Vaccination status	Sex					
	Male		Female		Total	P value
	Frequency	%	Frequency	%		
Vaccinated	204	83.6	179	86.9	383	0.33
Non-vaccinated	40	16.4	27	13.1	67	
Total	244	100	306	100	450	

Table 2.
The coverage of hepatitis B vaccination among 5-8 year-old children in Addis Ababa.

3.2 Vaccination status

383 (85.1%) out of 450 children had received HBV vaccination, of which 99.2% (380/383) of them had received the complete three doses of the vaccination. Only two (0.8%) children among the vaccinated had taken just two doses of the vaccine. There was no one who took only a single dose of the vaccine. The proportion of girls vaccinated (86.9%) is slightly higher than of boys (83.6%) as tabulated in **Table 2**.

3.3 Level of anti HBsAg Ab

Anti-HBsAg concentration > 10mIU/ml was observed in 214 (47.6%) children, six of whom were unvaccinated. Among the 383 vaccinated children, 208 (54.3%) had a protective level of antibody concentration (anti-HBsAg concentration of >10mIU/ml), while the remaining 47.3% did not. Among 67 unvaccinated children, 61 (91%) had anti HBsAg <10mIU/ml. From the three HIV infected participants, two of them were vaccinated. However, they did not have protective level antibody response (anti-HBsAg <10mIU/ml) (**Figure 1**).

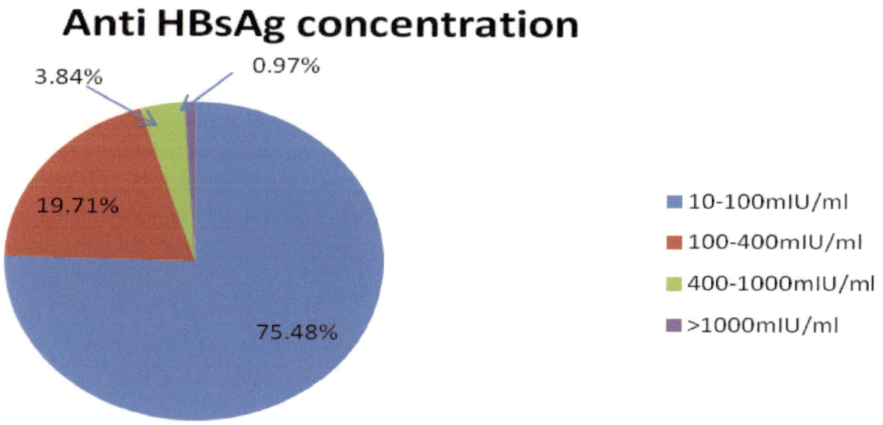

Figure 1.
Antibody response against hepatitis B vaccine in children between 5 and 8 years, Addis Ababa Ethiopia.

Variables	Categories	Number (n)	Percent (%)	P value
Sex	Male	15(244)	6.1	0.551
	Female	10(196)	4.9	
Vaccination status	Vaccinated	10(383)	2.6	0.000
	Not vaccinated	15(67)	22.4	
Age	5	4(95)	4.2	0.03
	6	3(130)	2.3	
	7	5(124)	4.0	
	8	13(101)	12.9	
Previous disease status	Yes	5(66)	7.6	0.438
	No	20(384)	5.2	

Table 3.
Seroprevalence of anti-HBc in 5-8 years old children in Addis Ababa, 2016-2017.

Anti-HBsAg concentration by age: A protective level antibody response against HBV vaccine was observed in 52.6%, 60%, 43.5% and 37.1% of children at the ages of 5, 6, 7, and 8, respectively. There was a significant association between age and the concentration of anti-HBsAg ($p = 0.001$). The levels of antibody concentration decreased as the age of the participant increased.

Seroprevalence of hepatitis B: From 450 children, only two (0.4%) were positive for HBsAg and 25 (5.6%) were positive for anti-HBc. 1 child (0.2%) was positive for both HBsAg and anti-HBc (**Table 3**). The two children who were positive for HBsAg were females, 5 years old, asymptomatic, and vaccinated for HBV.

Among anti-HBc positive children, 15 (6.1%) were male while 10 (4.9%) were female. There was no significant association between sex and anti-HBcAb ($p = 0.551$). Ten (2.6%) of anti-HBc positive children had received vaccination prior to this study. Among non-vaccinated children in this study, 15 (22.4%) were anti-HBc positive. There was a negative correlation between vaccination status and anti- HBc positivity ($p = 0.000$).

The seroprevalence of anti-HBc was 4.2%, 2.3%, 4% and 12.9% in 5, 6, 7 and 8 year old children, respectively. Age was significantly associated with anti- HBc seroprevalence ($p = 0.03$).

4. Discussion

The primary goal of vaccination against HBV is to generate an effective antibody response against the virus. The efficacy of HBV vaccine has not been determined in Ethiopia since its introduction in 2007. HBV vaccine coverage rate observed (85.1%) in our study is comparable with the estimated (86%) national coverage reported in 2015 [6]. Evidence has shown that the immune response against the vaccine decreases with increasing age. Our study observed a similar association between age and immune response against HBV vaccine.

In this study, 54.3% of vaccinated children had protective antibody response, as well as was obtained with low seroprevalence of HBsAg and anti-HBc of 0.4% and 5.6%, respectively. This result is comparable with a study conducted in Yemen and in Iran, where 54.8% and 56.3% of the children had protective antibody responses, respectively [8, 9].

However, in other areas, higher proportions of children were reported with protective level antibody responses in comparison to our study. Studies con- ducted in different areas of Iran observed that 78% of 5-10 years old children [10], 84% of 5 to 7 years old children [11], and 87.6% of under 7 years old children [12] had a protective level antibody response against HBV. A study that was conducted in Spain also revealed that 85% of children at the age of seven had protective level antibody response to the vaccine [13]. The difference in these countries could be attributed to differences in dose, vaccine type, and vaccination route.

In contrast to our study, a lower proportion of children with protective level antibody responses were observed in other studies. For example, in a study conducted in Egypt, 39.3% of the children (6-12 years old) had protective level antibody responses [14]. In addition, in different areas of Iran, only 47.9% of 10-11 year old children [15], 48% of 7 to 9 year old children [16], and 30% of the 8 months to 15-year-old children [17] had between ages of 8 months and 15 years had protective level antibody responses against HBV vaccine. These differences may be due to sampling difference, type of vaccine, and different age for vaccine administration.

Seroprevalence of HBsAg among vaccinated children varies in different countries ranging from 0 to 2.5%. Seroprevalence of HBsAg was 1.8% in Yemen [8], 0.13% in Nepal [18], 2.3% in Papua New Guinea [19], 0.77% in Eastern China [20],

2.5% in northwest China [21], while it was 0.4% in our study. This difference in seroprevalence of HBV infection could be attributed to the difference in vaccine coverage and difference in vaccination schedule.

In our study, seroprevalence of anti-HBc was 5.6%, which is lower than anti-HBc seroprevalence observed in studies conducted in Gambia (17.7%) [22], China (14.1%) [21] and Iran (7.5%) [23]. These discrepancies in anti-HBc seroprevalence could be attributed to age difference, race, prevalence of HBV, and immune response level.

Nowadays, mutant hepatitis B viruses are spreading globally. Vaccination regime and vaccine type should also be considered when we administer the vaccine to the child. High seroprevalence of anti- HBc in vaccinated children may indicate the presence of an occult HBV infection, which is a concern for everyone that needs to be addressed [24].

4.1 Limitations of the study

Some children did not come with their vaccination card. Therefore, we had to use the words of their parents/guardians as evidence for vaccination, which is not always reliable. Other serological markers of active HBV infection, like HBeAg, were not examined in this study. Further, there was an unequal number of vaccinated and non-vaccinated children and the study design did not account for occult infections.

5. Conclusion and recommendation

The vaccine coverage observed in this study is similar to that of the national estimate in 2014. However, less than half of the children had a protective level of anti- body response against HBV vaccine. Further, a negative association between anti-HBsAg antibody concentration and age was observed. Serological markers for hepatitis B virus were low: 0.4% for HBsAg and 5.6% of anti-HBc.

Persistence of anti-HBs antibodies is necessary for the long-term protection against hepatitis B virus infection. Even if different factors can contribute to low antibody response against the vaccine, we need to follow up children after vaccination, in order to see the effect of the vaccine in producing the desired response over time.

Finally, further studies should be undertaken to determine the duration of antibody response against HBV vaccine that may help in which years the vaccine response becomes less and less. For those who did not respond to the vaccine, booster doses should be given to enhance immunological responses to the vaccine. This can be important to elevate the vaccine response. Follow up is needed for those children who are administered with booster doses to evaluate response against the vaccine in those children.

Acknowledgements

The Ministry of Health through the Clinical Research Capacity Building program at the Armauer Hansen Research Institute (AHRI) funded this study; therefore, we would like to extend our deepest gratitude to both institutions. We would also like to express our deepest appreciation to AHRI laboratory staff, study participants, health extension workers, and all others who supported us in every step of this work.

Conflict of interest

There was no conflict of interest among the authors or with any other parties.

Author details

Habtamu Biazin Kebede* and Seifegebriel Teshome
Department of Microbiology, Immunology and Parasitology, College of Health Sciences, Addis Ababa University, Ethiopia

*Address all correspondence to: habtamu.biazin@aau.edu.et

References

[1] WHO. Fact sheets, Hepatitis B. Accessed on October 9, 2018. Available from: URL: http://www.who.int/news-room/fact-sheets/detail/hepatitis-b. 2018.

[2] Gao S, Duan ZP, Coffin CS. Clinical relevance of hepatitis B virus variants. World J Hepatol. 2015;7(8):1086-1096

[3] WHO. Global Alert and Response. Hepatitis B. Prevention and treatment. Accessed by July 2, 2015. Available from: URL: http://www.who.int/csr/disease/hepatitis/ whocdscsrlyo20022/ en/index5.html 2002.

[4] WHO. Global immunization coverage. www.who.int/immunization/newsroom/ Global_immunization data October 2006.pdf.

[5] Françoisa G, Dochezb C, Mphahlelec MJ, Burnettd R, VanHala G, Meheus A. Hepatitis B vaccination in Africa: mission accomplished? The South Afri J Epid and Infect. 2008;**23**(1):24-28

[6] Ethiopia: WHO and UNICEF estimate of immunization coverage: 2015 revision, Available onURL:http//www.data.unicef.org. Accessed on July 2016.

[7] Franco E, Bagnato B, Marino MG, Meleleo C, Serino L, Zaratti L. Hepatitis B: Epidemiology and preven- tion in developing countries. World J Hepatol 2012; 4(3): 74-80.

[8] Al-Shamahy HA, Hanash SH, Rabbad IA, Al-Madhaji NM, Naser SM. Hepatitis B Vaccine Coverage and the Immune Response in Children under ten years old in Sana'a. Yemen: *SQU Med J*. 2011;**11**(1):77-82

[9] Norouzirad R, Shakurnia AH, Assarehzadegan MA, Serajian A, Khabazkhoob M. Serum Levels of Anti- Hepatitis B Surface Antibody among Vaccinated Population Aged 1 to 18 Years in Ahvaz City Southwest of Iran. Hepat Mon. 2014;**14**(1):1-5

[10] Rezaei M, Nooripoor S, Ghorbani R, Ramezanshams F, Mamishi S, Mahmoudi S. Seroprotection after hepatitis B vaccination in children aged 1 to 15 years in central province of Iran, Semnan. J PMH. 2014;**55**:1-3

[11] Yazdanpanah B, Safari M, Yazdanpanah S. Persistence of HBV Vac•cine's Protection and Response to Hepatitis B Booster Immuniza•tion in 5- to 7-Year-Old Children in the Kohgiloyeh and Boyerah•mad Province. Iran. Hepat Mon. 2010;**10**(1):17-21

[12] Esmaili M, Seyedkolal F. Evaluation of anti HBS levels in vacci•nated children against Hepatitis B, Amirkola Hospital, Babol. KAUMS J (FEYZ). 2003;**6**(4):45-49

[13] Gonzalez ML, Gonzalez JB, Salva F, Lardinois RA. 7-year follow-up of newborns vaccinated against hepatitis B. Vaccine. 1993;**11**:1033-1036

[14] Shaaban FA, Hassanin AI, Samy SM, Salama SI, Said ZN. Long term immunity to hepatitis B among a sample of fully vaccinated children in Cairo. Egypt. East Med Helth J. 2007;**13**(4):750-757

[15] Jafarzadeh A, Montazerifar SJ. Persistence of anti-HBs antibody and immunological memory in children vaccinated with hepatitis B vaccine at birth. J Ayub Med Coll Abbottabad. 2006;**18**:4-9

[16] Rafizade B, Kazemi AN, Amir Moghadami HR, MoosaviNasab N. Survey of Anti-HBs Serum Level in Vaccinated 7-9 Year-old Chil•dren in Zanjan City 2004. ZUMS J. 2004;**12**(47):49-55

[17] Aghakhani A, Banifazl M, Izadi N, McFarland W, Sofian M, Khadem-Sadegh A, et al. Persistence of an- tibody to hepatitis B surface antigen among vaccinated children in a low hepatitis B virus endemic area. World J Pediatr. *2011*;**7**(4):358-360

[18] Upreti SR, Gurung S, Patel M, Dixit SM, Krause LK, Shakya G, et al. Prevalence of chronic hepatitis B virus infection before and after implementation of a hepatitis B vaccination program among children in Nepal. Vaccine. 2014;**32**(34):4304-4309

[19] Kitau R, Datta SS, Minal K. Patel MK, Hennessey K, Wannemuehler K et al. Hepatitis B Surface Antigen Seroprevalence among Children in Papua New Guinea, 2012-2013. Am. J. Trop. Med. *Hyg* 2015;92(3): 501-506

[20] Huang P, Zhu LG, Zhu YF, Yue M, Su J, Zhu FC, et al. Seroepidemiology of hepatitis B virus infection and impact of vaccination. World J Gastroenterol. 2015;**21**(25):7842-7850

[21] Ji Z, Wang T, Shao Z, Huang D, Wang A, Guo Z et al. A Population-Based Study Examining Hepatitis B Virus Infection and Immunization Rates in Northwest China. PLoS ONE 2014: 9(5).

[22] Van der Sande MAB, Waight PA, Mendy M, Zaman S, Kaye S, Sam O et al Long-Term Protection against HBV Chronic Carriage of Gambian Adolescents Vaccinated in Infancy and Immune Response in HBV Booster Trial in Adolescence. PLoS ONE 2007; 2(8): e753.

[23] Jafarzadeh A, Montazerifar SJ. Persistence of anti-HBs antibody and immunological memory in children vaccinated with hepatitis B vaccine at birth. J Ayub Med Coll Abbottabad. 2006;**18**:4-9

[24] Zeinab NAS. An overview of occult hepatitis B virus infection. World J Gastroenterol. 2011;**17**(15):1927-1938

Section 4

Safe Blood Transfusion in Beta-Thalassemia

Chapter 5

Novel Diagnostic Approach and Safe Blood Transfusion Practices for Thalassemia: A Vital Role of a Blood Centre in Western India

Avani Shah, Sumit Bharadva, Parizad Patel and Kanchan Mishra

Abstract

β-Thalassemia carrier's frequency is uneven in different districts in Gujarat (0–9.5%). Surat Raktadan Kendra & Research Centre (SRKRC), NABH accredited and regional blood Centre in Surat (Gujarat, India) running since 1976, provides free blood units to more than 350 Thalassemia Major Patients every year. Our DSIR (Department of Scientific and Industrial Research, Ministry of Science and Technology, Govt. of India) approved Research department has developed Multiplex ARMS-PCR including 4 common mutations which is a fast, reliable, and cost-effective method. Safe blood transfusion is a priority for these patients because of having transfusion-associated infections, formation of alloantibodies against donor's antigens, developing different grades of Blood Transfusion Reactions (BTR's), etc. Therefore, different approaches have been implemented as routine practice by our Blood Centre, like the use of saline washed and/or leuco-reduced Red Cell Concentrate for transfusion (reduces the risk of BTR's), NAT testing for Transfusion Transmitted Infections (reduces window period of TTI's), antibody screening of patient (if develop in patient) and molecular genotyping of clinically important blood group antigens (Difficult to type these patients serologically due to presence of donors' red cells). Despite being Blood Centre, contributing to developing novel diagnostic techniques and strictly following all possible transfusion practices, SRKRC greatly helps in ensuring proper diagnosis, lengthening the transfusion period and providing the safest blood to these patients.

Keywords: β-Thalassemia in India, multiplex ARMS-PCR, NAT testing, molecular genotyping, blood transfusion, alloantibodies

1. Introduction

From a historical perspective, it is always a question and debate in what way β-thalassemia has spread in the world to reach such high incidences in certain populations. Hemoglobinopathies, including hemoglobin variants and thalassemia, are a group of inherited disorders that arise due to mutation and/or deletions of one or more globin genes that result in the production of structurally abnormal Hb variants in the former and reduced rate of synthesis of the normal globin chains in the latter [1, 2]. Thalassemia is a group of disorders of hemoglobin in which either globin chain synthesis is reduced or absent, therefore it is termed as a quantitative disorder [3]. This inherited disorder of hemoglobin is considered the commonest single-gene disorder globally with an autosomal recessive inheritance, which estimated around 300,000 to 400,000 babies born each year suffering from the same [4]. It is increasingly prevalent in the Mediterranean, Asia and Sub-Saharan Africa along with other continents such as Europe, North America, and Australia due to population migration and therefore, has become a global health problem [5]. The carrier frequencies for β-thalassemia in these areas range from 1 to 20%, and rarely may be higher. The frequencies for the milder forms of β-thalassemia are much greater, varying from 10 to 20% in parts of sub- Saharan Africa to 40% or more in some Middle Eastern and Indian populations, to as high as 80% in northern Papua New Guinea and some isolated groups in the northeast of India [4].

1.1 The hemoglobinopathies: Burden in India

Among the different hemoglobinopathies, Beta-thalassemias and Sickle Cell Disorders (SCD) pose a significant health burden in India. The average prevalence of β-thalassemia carriers is 3–4%, which translates to 35 to 45 million carriers in our multi-ethnic and culturally and linguistically diverse population of 1.21 billion people that also includes around 8% of tribal groups. Several ethnic groups have a much higher prevalence (4–17%) [6, 7]. Every year 10,000 children are being born with thalassemia which approximately accounts for 10% of the total world incidence of thalassemia-affected children [8] and one in eight thalassemia carriers live in India. There are nearly 42 million carriers of the β-thalassemia trait. There are communities in which it is more prevalent like Sindhis, Punjabis, Gujaratis, Bengalis, Mahars, Kolis, Saraswats, Lohanas, and Gaurs [9]. However, in the absence of National Registries of patients, the exact numbers are not known. The March of Dimes Global Report on Birth Defects has estimated that the prevalence of pathological hemoglobinopathies in India is 1.2 per 1000 live births. It has been suggested that there would be 32,400 babies with a serious hemoglobin disorder born each year based on 27 million births per year in India [10–12]. Of the 10,000 to 12,000 thalassemic children born annually in India, very few are optimally managed mainly in urban regions although the Government of India has included the care and management of patients with thalassemia and sickle cell disease in the 12th Five Year Plan. It has been estimated that 2 million units of packed red cells would be needed for transfusion of thalassemia patients in the country [13, 14]. Better management for beta-thalassemia major patients mainly in urban regions in India with regular and safe blood transfusions and adequate iron chelation allows them to have a better quality of life.

Hemoglobinopathies are more common in Gujarat compared to other Indian states. Model and Petrou [15] have estimated a 12% incidence of major hemoglobinopathy traits in Gujarat. Several studies have revealed a high prevalence of β-thalassemia trait (BTT) in some caste groups in Gujarat [16–18]. Certain castes and tribes in Gujarat are yet to be investigated for thalassemia and other abnormal haemoglobins. About 10–15% of the tribal population of India is in Gujarat, particularly in South Gujarat and the prevalence of sickle cell trait (SCT) varies from 0 to 31.4% among different tribes [19, 20].

2. Counseling, screening and prevention of beta-thalassemia

Diagnosis and management of this disorder both in adults and in newborns, using appropriate approaches and uniform technology are important in different regions of a vast and diverse country like India. SRKRC is running a screening and prevention program for Beta-thalassemia and Sickle cell anemia for the last 15 years. Under this program, students from colleges and universities are screened for hemoglobinopathies. The prevalence of Beta-thalassemia trait (BTT) was 4.4% and sickle cell anemia was 1.3%, reported by SRKRC [20]. Castes like Lohana (10.8%), Sindhi (10.2%), Prajapati (6.3%) and Ghanchi (6.2%) had a higher prevalence of BTT, whereas Gamit, Vasava, Chaudhary and Mahyavanshi had a higher prevalence of BTT (15.9, 13.6, and 6.9%) and SCT (22.2, 15.2, and 4.2%) respectively [20]. This prevalence rate is not much different from the other parts of the country. Surat is a multiethnic city. Castes like Lohana, Sindhi, Prajapati, Ghanchi, Gamit, Vasava, Chaudhary, and Mahyavanshi have a high prevalence of thalassemia and sickle cell anemia are prevalent. In Surat city, the prevalence of Beta- thalassemia trait was 4.4% and sickle cell anemia was 1.3%, reported by SRKRC.

2.1 Counseling for hemoglobinopathies

In every part of the world, there are individual groups that require counseling for screening and diagnosis of their disease status. Such groups are [21];

- Pre-marriage counseling and screening
- Antenatal screening
- Preconception counseling and screening
- Prenatal diagnosis
- Neonatal screening
- Cord Blood for Haemoglobinopathy Screening
- Genetic counseling

2.1.1 Pre-marriage counseling and screening

Undiagnosed Hemoglobinopathies is a potential threat, pre-marriage counseling and screening is quick way that brings immediate change and result. In India still, 50% of the marriages take place where a girl and a boy do not know each other. In such premarital counseling can be difficult. Premarital counseling can be done after screening the carrier state of an individual and making him/her understand the importance of this test and future consequences. Counseling can be done by preparing booklets, short movies and posters to increase awareness in society. The marriage register can also do premarital consoling when any marriage gets registered at the marriage registrar's office. In villages, the main leaders or panchayatmukhiya can take the responsibility of counseling and increase awareness among the people. Furthermore, some studies found the increased rate of marriage cancelation due to a better understanding of the disease and counseling by the couples at risk [22]. However, the actual targets have not been achieved yet due to many reasons including consanguineous marriages, screening just before the marriage, individual or family commitment, non-availability of alternative suitable partner, etc.

2.1.2 Antenatal screening

It is very important in cases where premarital testing has not been done. Antenatal screening usually takes place roughly between 12- and 20-weeks gestations of pregnancy. This screening is a sandwich between premarital screenings, counseling and prenatal diagnosis. After the antenatal screening, if both the partners found minor for Beta- thalassemia or sickle cell anemia, proper counseling should be done for prenatal diagnosis. When a thalassemia major child takes birth, to give him/her quite healthy and stable life a family needs to bear almost 2 lakhs per year including blood transfusion and medications. Even after spending such a huge amount of money and other pain full procedures of blood transfusion, a major child may not live more than 20–30 yrs. We can prevent the birth of such a child with the help of prenatal diagnosis by spending 10,000 rupees. By preventing the birth of a thalassemia major child, we can get rid of pain and disappointment.

2.1.3 Preconception counseling and screening

The infertility rate has increased due to stress, unhealthy lifestyles, marriages at older age, etc. that ultimately enhances procedures like Intra-Uterine Insemination (IUI) and In-vitro Fertilization (IVF). Both these procedures should be done under the medical council guidelines. However, in India, it is very difficult where even pregnant women do not register in clinics before 12 weeks of gestation. In the case of preconception, counseling and screening are very important as if anyone partner is minor; another partner of egg/sperm donor must be screened for the same before conception.

2.1.4 Prenatal diagnosis

The purpose of prenatal hemoglobinopathy screening is to identify and counsel asymptomatic individuals whose offspring are at risk of an inherited hemoglobinopathy. Although, prenatal diagnosis is a huge set-up and sustains process that needs expertise in molecular biology techniques. Proper and effective counseling is the key factor for prenatal diagnosis. A couple who are not screened for Beta-thalassemia minor and diagnosed at the time of pregnancy, for such kind of couple would be requiring prenatal diagnosis within 3 months of pregnancy. After the result of prenatal diagnosis, if the unborn is diagnosed as thalassemia major, a gynecologist may give an option of abortion to such a couple.

2.1.5 Neonatal screening

Universal screening should be done where all newborn babies in these high-risk groups are screened, as this would allow identification of other clinically significant disorders such as homozygous Beta-thalassemia and all cases of Hb S–Beta-thalassemia that could be transfusion dependent. Minor couples who do not go for prenatal diagnosis, their newborn should be tested for mutation of thalassemia major.

2.1.6 Genetic counseling

Once a thalassemia major baby is born in a family it is very important to make the parents and the family understands the consensus of the disease. Genetic guidance is an effective preventive and educational process that improved the quality of life of patients, preventing complications and sequels and allowed the referral of those who may transmit altered genes for clinical diagnosis and to genetic counseling services. A trained counselor, a hematologist or a pediatrician can effectively do this job. It is always a challenge for a family to raise such a diseased child like a normal one, moreover to bear the mental, physical and economical trauma lifelong that will be associated with the blood transfusions and other treatments for the child.

2.2 Methodologies for Hemoglobinopathy screening and diagnosis: guidelines for laboratories

For screening and detection of hemoglobinopathies especially the minor cases, certain guidelines have been prepared nationally and internationally [21, 23–28]. In India, the Ministry of Health and Welfare, Government of India issued "Guidelines on hemoglobinopathies in India" in the year 2016 [28]. Before screening test, individuals' family history, clinical evaluation if any, family origin, basic details like age, birth date, gender, the occupation should be recorded in the form of informed consent. A basic test like complete blood count (CBC) on an automated or semi-automated analyzer along with the stained peripheral blood smear should be assessed primarily. Abnormal red cell morphologies like microcytosis, iron deficiency anemia and anemia of chronic disease should be ruled out and investigations would be carried out for thalassemia with considering other hemoglobinopathies as well.

An automated cation exchange High-Performance Liquid Chromatography (HPLC) is the method of choice for hemoglobin estimation. HPLC gives an accurate estimation and quantification of different haemoglobins (Hb) like Hb A2, Hb F, Hb A and also the detection of Hb variants like HbS, HbD, HbE, HbD Punjab, etc. Despite the high cost of HPLC machines, many centres in India have this facility. The accuracy of HPLC is very high than that of the electrophoresis processes which is a more manual method compared to HPLC. Methods like isoelectric focusing, capillary and paper electrophoresis were earlier choices to use, now not used extensively in India. Followings are the screening tests used for thalassemia and other hemoglobinopathies.

2.2.1 Naked eye single tube red cell osmotic fragility test (NESTROFT)

This test is based on the osmotic fragility of red blood cells (RBCs) using the 0.36% buffered saline and has been used as a preliminary test particularly for the Beta-thalassemia carriers in India. The excessive use of this test in India may be because of the low cost, no need for any specialized equipment, and result within 10 minutes though the test gives false results due to very low specificity, false positivity, and false negativity in many clinical conditions like iron deficiency anemia where RBCs become fragile. Especially it is not recommended where automated cell counters are available. However, the primary investigation of large population in the rural area with fewer facilities would be carried out with this test.

2.2.2 Red blood cell indices- complete blood count (CBC)

There are substantial changes are happening in the RBC indices in the case of Beta-thalassemia minor with Mean corpuscular volume (MCV) <80 fl and Mean corpuscular hemoglobin concentration (MCH) <27 pg. with usually high RBC counts for the level of hemoglobin. Deviations in indices occur when samples are not run within a few hours. In such a case MCH is a more stable and reliable parameter than MCV. It is not always the case that each Beta-thalassemia minor has low MCV, MCH and high RBC count, Atypical Beta-thalassemia minor may show completely normal indices which can be missed during screening.

2.2.3 Quantization of HbA2

Hb A2 levels >4.0% along with low MCV, MCH and higher RBC counts are considered as the classical case of Beta-thalassemia carrier. HPLC being the method of choice gives an accurate quantification of Hb A2. Correct interpretations of borderline HbA2 levels (3.3–3.9%) are of utmost importance and need to be done with great caution. Such borderline cases should be confirmed by the DNA-based diagnostic methods. Mutations in the promoter region or the poly-A tail of the b-globin gene may have the completely normal RBC indices and/or HbA2 in the Beta-thalassemia carriers. **Figures 1** and **2** depict the retention time graph of different hemoglobins on HPLC (Figures obtained from our Research department).

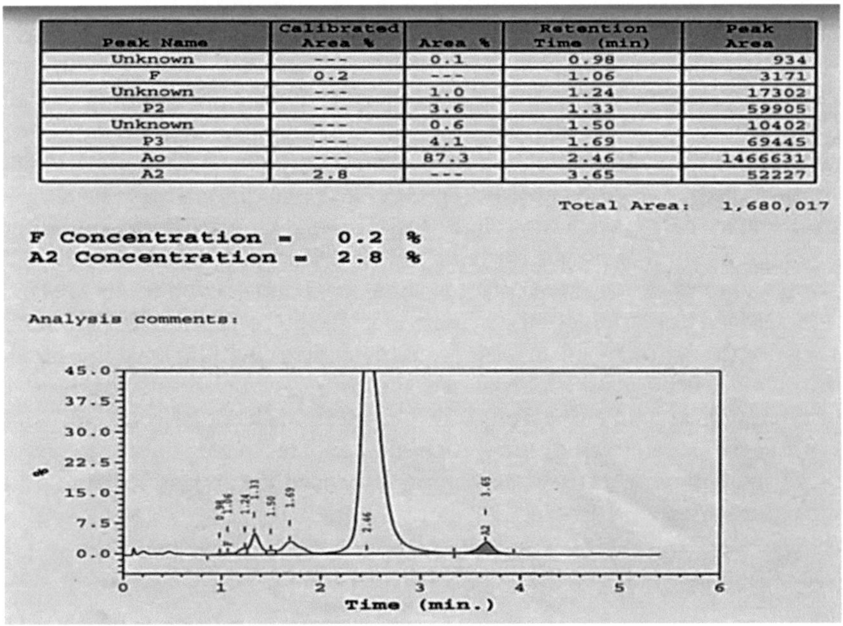

Peak Name	Calibrated Area %	Area %	Retention Time (min)	Peak Area
Unknown	---	0.1	0.98	934
F	0.2	---	1.06	3171
Unknown	---	1.0	1.24	17302
P2	---	3.6	1.33	59905
Unknown	---	0.6	1.50	10402
P3	---	4.1	1.69	69445
Ao	---	87.3	2.46	1466631
A2	2.8	---	3.65	52227

Total Area: 1,680,017

F Concentration = 0.2 %
A2 Concentration = 2.8 %

Analysis comments:

Figure 1.
HPLC report of with normal levels of Hb A2.

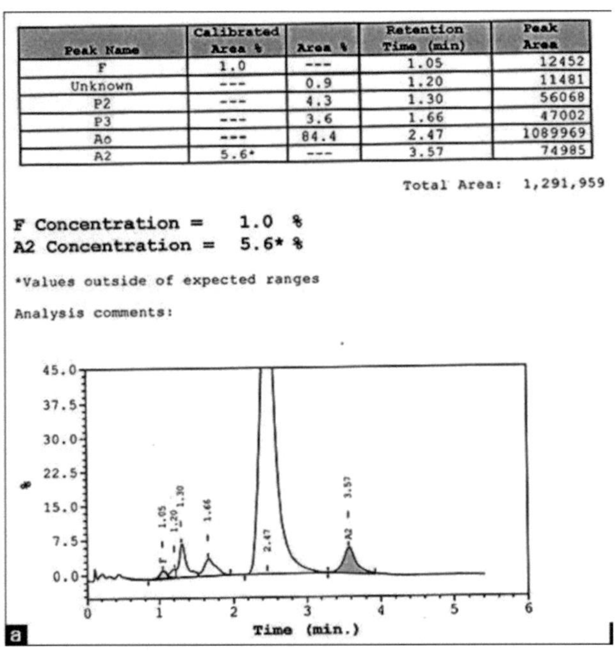

Peak Name	Calibrated Area %	Area %	Retention Time (min)	Peak Area
F	1.0	---	1.05	12452
Unknown	---	0.9	1.20	11481
P2	---	4.3	1.30	56068
P3	---	3.6	1.66	47002
Ao	---	84.4	2.47	1089969
A2	5.6*	---	3.57	74985

Total Area: 1,291,959

F Concentration = 1.0 %
A2 Concentration = 5.6* %

*Values outside of expected ranges

Analysis comments:

Figure 2.
HPLC report of high levels of Hb A2: A case of Beta-thalassemia.

Quantification of other hemoglobin variants apart from Hb A2 is also important to know the heterozygosity with two Hb variants like Beta-thalassemia carriers + sickle cell anemia carriers, Beta-thalassemia carriers + Hb E carriers, Beta-thalassemia carriers + Hb D carriers, etc. HPLC results with >10%, HbA2% is suggestive of the presence of other Hb variants like HPLC also quantifies Hb S, Hb D Punjab and Hb E and some fewer common variants which may elute in the P3 window (Hb J variants) or as unknown peaks.

Many large studies, either hospital-based or population screening programs for identification of hemoglobinopathies using HPLC analysis have been reported from India recently [12–14, 25, 29–32]. A multicenter study on screening university students and pregnant women in six states (Maharashtra, Gujarat, Karnataka, West Bengal, Assam, and Punjab) showed that the prevalence of Beta-thalassemia varied from 1.48% to 3.64% [12].

A large study on screening for hemoglobinopathies among non-tribal and tribal populations from different cities in Gujarat showed an overall prevalence of Beta-thalassemia trait of 1.95% and HbS trait of 6.5%. A high prevalence of Beta-thalassemia trait was seen among the Bhanushalis (8.1%), Bhakta (7.9%) and Lohanas (6.5%) [20]. A study of 65,779 cases by HPLC from Maharashtra reported 11.2% of BTT and 2.2% of SCT [33]. Tribal groups in Maharashtra have shown a prevalence of the Beta-thalassemia trait of 1.6 to 5.6% [34] while the prevalence of Beta-thalassemia trait has also been high (6.3 to 8.5%) among some tribal groups in Orissa [35] and in the non-tribal populations of Madhya Pradesh in Central India (9.59%) [36]. Thus, Beta-thalassemia is not uncommon among many non-tribal and tribal populations in India.

2.2.4 Cellulose acetate electrophoresis

This is completely a manual technique starting from preparing the hemolysate to the quantifying bands that appear on the cellulose acetate membrane at alkaline pH. Such manual technique required adequate experience and high skills. The technique is not used at those centres where HPLC is available as it's a manual, time-consuming and cumbersome method and results may vary from person to person though it is highly cost-effective compared to HPLC.

2.2.5 Quantization of Hb F

Quantification of Hb F (Fetal hemoglobin) is extremely important to identify diseased and carrier conditions. HPLC is one of the most widely used methods for this purpose. Earlier alkali denaturation was extensively used for the same. Hb F is the important parameter for the Indian population to differentiate between Beta-thalassemia and iron deficiency anemia because later is also more prevalent in India. When Hb F is being enumerated using HPLC, it needs to be ensured that the peak coming into the Hb F window is Hb F and not another Hb variant. **Figure 3** shows the diagrammatic view of screening carrier cases of hemoglobinopathies.

2.2.6 Molecular methods for the confirmation of mutations

Common Polymerase Chain Reaction (PCR) based detection techniques used for identifying the Beta-thalassemia point mutations are allele-specific PCR, reverse dot blot (RDB) analysis, real-time PCR with melting curve analysis, and DNA sequencing [28, 37]. DBS (Dried blood spot) filter paper matrix is required for the extraction of DNA from the whole blood sample which includes crude boiling preparation, alkali denaturation and other kit-based methods. As per the laboratory

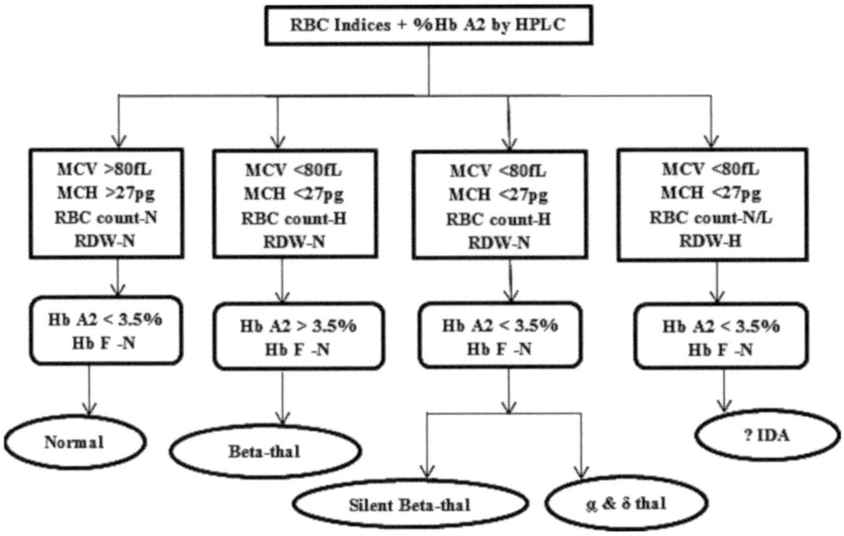

Figure 3.
Screening of Beta-thalassemia carriers and other haemoglobinopathies [37].

need and setup, the best methods of DNA extraction for PCR-based analysis may be selected [38]. PCR-based molecular assays are extremely susceptible to the aerosol contamination of amplicons. To minimize this one way-directional workflow is required that is amplification and analysis must be done in the separated rooms/labs with all the necessary and safety precautions [39]. A positive control (having genotype positive DBS or known samples for heterozygous or homozygous hemoglobinopathies), negative control and a regent control (no template control) must be run with each PCR protocol.

2.2.6.1 Allele-specific PCR

This technique employs two primers identical in sequence except for the 30- terminus base, one of which is complementary to the wild type and the other for the mutant base; a common primer for the opposite strand must of course be used as well [37]. For primer extension to occur using Taq polymerase which has no 30–50 exonuclease (proofreading) activity, perfect matching of the primer 30-terminus with the DNA template must occur. With a normal individual, the PCR product will be seen only in the reaction employing the wild-type primer set. A heterozygote will generate a band using both wild type and mutant primer set, and an individual with a homozygous mutation will be negative with the normal and positive with the mutant primer set.

2.2.6.2 Reverse dot-blot hybridization

This is quite a routine procedure identifying suspected mutation using hybridization of an allele-specific oligomer (ASO) DNA probe [37]. For each mutation, two hybridization reactions are conducted, one with the probe for the mutant sequence and the normal sequence. The stringency of hybridization has to be optimized for each ASO probe. The ASO probes have an amino group at the 50-terminal base that enables them to attach to the nylon membrane strip after this hybridization takes place with amplified DNA that is labeled with biotin. Normal allele gives develop dots with each wild type probe but not with any mutant probe.

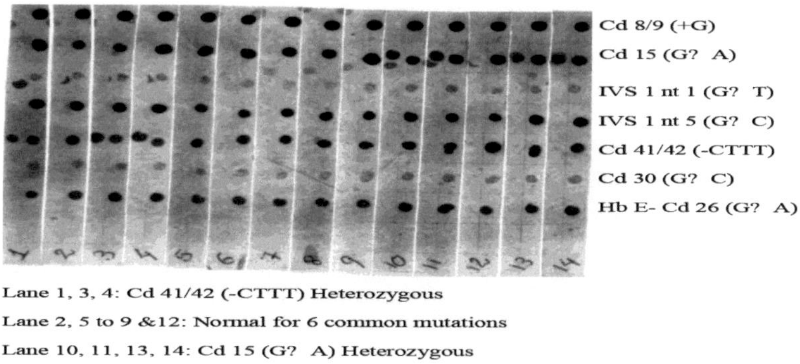

Figure 4.
Detection of common Indian Beta-globin gene mutation by CRDB (source: Obtained from in-house experiment).

Minor/carrier/heterozygotes give one mutation dot and one normal dot, whereas major/homozygotes give dot with the only mutated probe. Being a semi-automated method critical care should be taken at the time of washing the blots and optimization is required that can be achieved by the optimizing ASO probe length. **Figure 4** shows the in-house developed blots of different thalassemia mutations.

2.2.6.3 Novel approach: multiplex ARMS-PCR for detecting 4 common Beta-thalassemia mutations

The analysis of transfusion-dependent thalassemia major cases, attending our centre, suggested that there is a high prevalence in Muslims, Patels, Sindhis, ModhBanias, and Mahayavanshi [40–42]. Certain sub-castes of Patel [19] and tribal communities are already studied for sickle cell disorders [43, 44]. Dhodia Patel, the third largest tribal group in Gujarat, needs b-thalassemia studies as thalassemia major cases are identified in this community [41, 42].

The purpose of the present investigation was to establish and standardize a multiplex-ARMS procedure to detect ethnic-specific common mutations like IVS I-5 (G/C), Codon 41/42 (-TCTT), 619-bp deletion and FS 8/9 (þG) in one tube. This method is very convenient to screen the most commonly known molecular defects in a single Multiplex ARMS-PCR tube and detection on agarose gel electrophoresis based on specific PCR product size for each mutation [45–48].

Our in-house developed method was subsequently tested on 110 unrelated samples with unidentified Beta-thalassemia mutations. The codons IVS 1–5 mutation was the most common beta-thalassemia mutation in the Surat population. The following mutations were presented in decreasing frequency: IVS 1e5 (G/C) < Codon 8/9 (þG) < Codon 41/42 (-CTTT) < 619 bp deletion. **Figure 5** shows the amplification of 4 common mutations on an agarose gel stained with ethidium bromide. This ARMS multiplex system was found reliable, cost-effective, fast and most applicable for mutation screening of Thalassemia in Surat populations [40].

2.2.6.4 A comprehensive next-generation sequencing (NGS) platform for screening and genotyping in subjects with Hemoglobinopathies

The next advance in molecular diagnostics for hemoglobin disorders will be next-generation sequencing. Recently, NGS has been introduced to screen for thalassemia. More loci including genetic modifiers which have significant effects on clinical manifestation should be covered in the NGS screening, which is important for precise diagnosis and treatment of thalassemia [49–51].

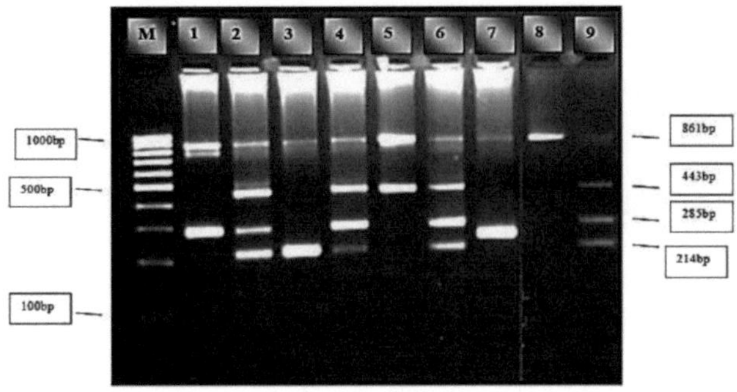

Figure 5.
3% agarose gel showing the multiplex ARMS-PCR for four common mutation of Beta-thalassemia.

There will be some technical challenges in implementing next-generation sequencing, especially for the HBA genes, which, because of the nearly identical sequence between the HBA1 and HBA2 genes, will make it challenging to determine whether a given mutation belongs to one or the other of these genes. We can hope that the cost of these technologies will eventually decrease enough to make them available to resource-limited settings where the diagnosis of hemoglobin disorders will be most valuable.

2.2.6.5 Other DNA based methods

Several other methods are used apart from these above-mentioned. In that Real-time PCR with melting curve analysis, Direct DNA sequencing, multiplex ligation-dependent probe amplification (MLPA) and Next-generation sequencing have been used. RT-PCR or quantitative PCR eliminates the post PCR steps, time consumption and labour intensiveness of conventional PCRs [52, 53]. If any novel or rare mutation is present in the population, direct DNA sequencing would be the best method for the same that uses streptavidin-coated magnetic beads [54, 55]. MLPA allows the detection of any deletions or duplications in the screened regions. It requires only thermocycler and CE equipment [30, 56]. Limitations of conventional thalassemia diagnosis methods are missed diagnoses due to normal or borderline red blood cell indices and/or Hb A2 levels, various labour-intensive methods may need to identify disease-causing mutation for thalassemia that have more than 1800 mutations ranging from point mutation to large deletion.

2.3 Prevention and control of Beta-thalassemia

2.3.1 Creating awareness in the general population

The success of the prevention and control of any disease depends upon the awareness among the general population and how well the population is educated about the same [57]. In India, many social welfare clubs like Rotary, Lions, various NGOs, even Thalassemia Parents-Patients societies have been conducting education and awareness programs. Yet, awareness about b thalassemia among pregnant women in 6 states in the multi-centric Jai Vigyan programme was very limited varying from 0.2% to 4.8% in Bangalore, Vadodara, Mumbai, Dibrugarh and Ludhiana and 20.7% in Kolkata [25]. More than 50% of the rural population has not heard about thalassemia or they have some misconceptions and myths regarding this [34], whereas the majority of the people of urban areas were not ready for pre-marital screening [35]. Yet thalassemia education has not been included in the high school curriculum in India. However, this strategy has worked in the Mediterranean region [6]. The use of mass media would create a great impact over a longer period by repeatedly showing the short films or programs on thalassemia [36].

2.3.2 Target population screening for prevention and control

For every country and population single strategy may not work all the time [28]. Defining and selecting the target population and their screening on time are the important aspects for possible prevention and control. **Table 1** shows the different timings and the age groups where screening can be possible.

3. Role of a blood center in the management of β-thalassemia patients

A Blood center plays a crucial role in providing safe blood particularly to those patients for whom RBC transfusion is the principal support to live. As stated by the World Health Organization (WHO), nearly 120 million units of blood are donated every year. However, this is not sufficient to meet the global need many patients requiring a transfusion do not have timely access to safe blood. Regular donations are required to ensure there is always a supply for those in need. Maintaining safe and effective procedures around the collection, storage and use of donated blood is essential. Collectively called haemovigilance, these procedures cover the entire blood transfusion chain and are used to standardize the use of blood in healthcare.

The Blood Transfusion Service (BTS) in India is fragmented and disintegrated under various controls, and there is a wide gap between demand and supply. As said by the Executive Director of Thalassaemia International Federation, India is a sub-continent with a population of 1,380,004,385 people (17.7 per cent of the total global population). It has an estimated prevalence of patients with Transfusion-Dependent β-Thalassaemia (TDT) of 150,000 with a predicted annual number of affected births of 12,500. With such a disease burden, there is a huge requirement for Blood centers and blood donors. Based on current estimates, an estimated two million units/year of packed red cells are needed to address the needs of TDT in India [58].

Target population	Screenig & probable preventive meassures
Newborn	• Suitable for screening for Sickle Cell Disease and few cases of Thalassemia major • Early and proper treatment would be started for controlling the disease condition
Adolescence	• Most suitable for carrier screening • Early prevention & control even before the time of marriage, if screened as carrier
Premarital	• Carrier screening at this stage is effective in a community • Like in adolescent, carrier-carrier marriage may be prevented as preventive measure
Antenatal screening/ Prenatal diagnosis (PND)/ Preconception	• If both parents are carriers i.e. “at-risk” couple: then the status of the fetus for Thalassemia disease or sickle cell disease can be ascertained through prenatal diagnosis. • After PND analysis, couple may abort the child which could be the best preventive & control measure

Table 1.
Population screening & preventive measures needs to be taken.

Indian Ministry of Health and Family Welfare (MoH& FW) identified 2626 functional Blood centers across the country in the year 2016 from which, 76 per cent were public and not-for-profit-owned and 24 per cent were owned by the private sector. However, 61 per cent of these were situated in eight states, out of which only two (Maharashtra and Gujarat) have a high thalassemia prevalence. The Blood centers/ million population in high thalassemia-prevalence states, including Uttar Pradesh (1.2), West Bengal (1.3), Rajasthan (1.5) and Chhattisgarh (two) is less than the national average of 2.2 Blood centers/1,000,000 population. It was estimated in 2017 that the annual collection was 11.1 million units of blood while the demand was 14.6 million units [58].

In Thalassemia Major Patient's transfusion therapy is often initiated before one or two years of age [59–62]. Complications directly related to transfusion include blood-borne infections, development of anti-RBC antibodies (both auto- and allo-immunization), and allergic, febrile or delayed hemolytic transfusion reactions. Hb levels above 12.0 g/dL for adult women and 13.0 g/dL for adult men are considered normal [63]. General transfusion guidelines recommend initiating transfusions at an Hb threshold of 6.0–10.0 g/L, depending on the presence and severity of clinical conditions [64]; however, these guidelines focus mainly on correcting anemia rather than suppressing ineffective erythropoiesis and may not be applicable to patients with β- thalassemia [65]. Guidelines for the management of β-thalassemia are available, including international guidelines by the Thalassaemia International Federation (TIF) [66, 67] and several national guidelines [68–70].

3.1 Guidelines for blood transfusion in Beta-thalassemia patients

Life-long and regular blood transfusion is required to treat thalassemia major. This results in excessive accumulation of iron in the body (iron overload) that in the long term gives severe clinical complications such as heart and liver failure, diabetes, hypogonadism. Iron overload may be prevented and treated by daily removal (iron chelation therapy) [71–73].

Patients with β-thalassaemia major should receive leucoreduced packed red blood cells with a minimum hemoglobin content of 40 g [66, 67]. Only the transfusion of pRBCs can maintain the required hemoglobin percentage necessary for the normal growth of the diseased child. The transfused blood should be obtained from voluntary non-paid donors and collected, processed, screened, stored and transported by a trusted and high-quality blood transfusion centre [59]. If possible fresh blood should be transfused (not older than 10–12 days) as 2, 3-DPG (2, 3-Di-phophoglyceric acid) gets depleted in stored blood that reducing the capacity to deliver oxygen to the tissues [74]. Decreased recovery and shortened half-life may increase transfusion requirements. For all these, it is important to strengthen the Blood centers and component therapy should be ensured and mandatory. As per the guideline issued by the Indian Ministry of Health & Welfare in the year 2016 [28], A blood centre should be fully occupied with good infrastructure having component separation facility without that packed red cells are not available, and pretesting strategies should be followed for such chronically transfused patients are;

- Forward and Reverse blood group typing for ABO and RhD [28]

- In newly diagnosed patients along with ABO & RhD, extended phenotyping at least for C, c, E, e, Kell and Duffy would be desired [26, 74–78]

- Allo-antibody screening at regular intervals is necessary. If an alloantibody is detected, the patient should be transfused with that particular antigen-negative blood [26, 28]

- Every 3 months, patients should be tested for virus serology to detect initiation of the transfusion-transmitted infections (HIV, Hepatitis B, Hepatitis C viruses) [26, 28, 79]
- Ideally the patient should receive NAT (Nucleic Acid Amplification Test) tested blood product as NAT offers the possibility to minimized the window period [26, 28]
- Precautions for grouping, cross-matching and transfusion should be applied to chronically transfused patients like any other recipient [26, 28].
- Avoid close relative blood transfusion in such patients [26, 28].

3.2 Role of blood Centre in maintaining the national guidelines for β-thalassemia patients

As mentioned above it's the huge responsibility of every blood center to provide safe blood to these chronically transfused patients. Flowing are the procedures that should be carried out at every blood centre for providing safe blood and managing such patients.

3.2.1 Blood donations, quality of blood and Donor's motivation

For the health of chronically transfused patients with thalassemia, a blood donor should be careful by keeping the criteria of regular voluntary and non-paid donors [26, 28, 79]. The process of donor selection is usually done through questionnaires. These questionnaires are prepared by considering the national need, resources, the prevalence of the transfusion-transmitted infections and also by adhering to the directions from the European Union (EU), World Health Organization (WHO), American Association of Blood centers (AABB). Quality of collected blood would be maintained by proper collection, testing, stored and distribution following all the quality-controlled procedures. The huge problem of low blood donation and blood supply is a lack of voluntary and non-paid donors. A public awareness campaign, including posters and an annual event to honor donors, was implemented to encourage voluntary and non-paid blood donors [80].

3.2.2 Leukoreduced packed red blood cells

Leucocyte-reduced red blood cells concentrate should be prepared by a method known to deplete leucocytes in the final component to less than $5x10^8$ when intended to prevent febrile reactions and to less than $5x10^6$ when it is required to prevent alloimmunization or CMV infection [26, 28, 71, 79, 81]. For achieving a level $< 5x10^6$, the use of a leucocytes filter is necessary. Reduction of leukocytes to $5x10^6$ is considered the critical threshold for eliminating adverse reactions attributed to contaminating white cells and for preventing platelet alloimmunization. Two types of preparation methods for Leucocyte depleted packed RBCs are;

- **Prestorage filtration**: is the process to remove white blood cells from the whole blood which is carried out with an in-line filter within 8 hours after blood collection. Using this technique very high-efficiency filtration is achieved with consistently low WBC residue and high red cell recovery. The removal of the WBCs before storage will prevent the accumulation of cytokines during storage that leads to a reduction in the number of FNHTRs. This leukoreduced whole blood is centrifuged to obtain packed red cells.

- **Bedside filtration**: This technique is used for filtering red cell concentrators (RCC) at the bedside which may not allow optimal quality control, as the techniques used for bedside filtration are highly variable. Red cell concentrates are prepared from stored whole blood by removing plasma and buffy coats.

3.2.3 Other specific products for Thalassemic patients

- **Washed red cells** may be most beneficial for thalassemic patients who have repeated severe allergic transfusion reactions or individuals with IgA (Immunoglobulin A) deficiency which can cause an anaphylactic reaction [28, 71, 79, 81]. Washing of the whole blood removes plasma proteins that contain antibodies that may target patients. Washing may be done by automated or manual technique and must be transfused within 24 hrs because storage is not. Therefore, wastage may be possible if the patient is not available for transfusion at the time product is prepared. If suspension in SAGM (Saline, Adenine, Glucose, Mannitol) after washing in closed circuit, 14 days shelf life should be considered. Washing usually does not result in adequate leukocyte reduction and, therefore, should be used in conjunction with filtration. Washing of red cell units may remove some erythrocytes from the transfusion product.

- **Cryopreserved (frozen) red cells** are derived from whole blood within 7 days of collection in which RBCs are frozen using glycerol as cryopreserved and stored at −60°C to −80°C. Such type of frozen component is mainly used to supply rare donor units for patients who have atypical red cell antibodies or do not have high-frequency red cell antigens. The shelf life of this product is 1–7 days depending upon preparation in an open or closed system and resuspended in SAGM. Around 20% of the donor cells are lost in this freezing process and due to short life possibility of wastage is there. The Euro Blood center in Amsterdam, the Netherlands, provides a wide variety of special blood types

- **Neocyte transfusions** are the use of younger red blood cells (YRBCs) which can be separated from old cells by density gradient centrifugation [82] that can help to achieve extension of the transfusion interval [83–87].

3.2.4 Amount of blood to be transfused

Packed red blood cells 15 ml/kg body weight, should be administered at the rate of 5 ml/kg/hr [28]. As per the pre-transfused hemoglobin level, 1–2 units of pRBCs may be required by patients. 3.5 ml/kg of pRBCs with around 60% HCT can raise hemoglobin by 1gm/dl.

3.2.5 Storage and transport of red cell units

Different anticoagulant solutions are used to store the blood products which prevent coagulation and store red cells without losing their metabolic activity [28, 71, 79, 81]. **Table 2** shows the list of anticoagulants that are commonly used. In thalassaemia major decreased recovery and a shortened red cell half-life may increase transfusion requirements and as a consequence the rate of transfusion iron loading, the current practice is to use red cells stored in additive solutions for less than two weeks. Blood units should preferably be transported in monitored insulated boxes which maintain a temperature of between 2 and 8°C.

Name of Anticoagulant	Shelf life
CPD (Citrate, Phosphate, Dextrose)	21
CP2D (Citrate, Phosphate 2, Dextrose)	21
CPDA-1 (Citrate, Phosphate, Dextrose, Adenine)	35
CPD, CP2D or CPDA-1 with Additive solution	42

Table 2.
Anticoagulants and their shelf life period.

The following data should be regularly recorded at each transfusion:

- Date of transfusion
- Time of initiation and time of completion of transfusion.
- Bag number of the blood unit transfused
- Weight/volume of packed cells transfused
- Patient demographics (height, weight, pre-transfusion Hb, blood group and other details)
- Clinically assess the size of liver and spleen
- Transfusion details of each patient to be entered into their transfusion card, to ensure proper database maintenance and traceability.

3.2.6 Compatibility testing and alloantibody detection

Every recipient should receive ABO & RhD type specific compatible whole blood or red blood cell components [26, 28, 71, 79, 81]. 'O' packed red cells should be transfused only when ABO type specific unit is absent. RhD positive recipients can receive either RhD positive or negative components. But RhD negative recipient should receive transfusion only of RhD donor; however, in reasonable circumstances, RhD positive unit may be transfused only when the receiver does not have the RhD antibodies. In the case where clinically significant atypical antibodies are detected, a negative unit particular for that antigen or least compatible unit should be transfused. When a patient is massively transfused within a period of 24 hrs, a fresh sample should be used for subsequent transfusions.

In the case of multitransfused patients like thalassemia major and sickle cell disease, blood transfusion should be done after the confirmed diagnosis. Before the first transfusion, patients should be typed for complete red cell genotyping that help to determine subsequent development allo-antibodies in such patients after repeated transfusion of different blood units. The development of multiple allo-antibodies is common in these patients [88]. Therefore, it is important to monitor the patient carefully and to give him/her particular antigens negative blood unit for transfusion. Anti-E, anti-C and anti-Kell alloantibodies are most common. However, 5–10% of patients present with alloantibodies against rare erythrocyte antigens or with warm or cold antibodies of unidentified specificity [79].

Even before embarking on transfusion therapy, patients should have been gone through extended blood group antigen typing at least for C, c, E, e, and Kell which would be beneficial to identify antibodies in case of alloimmunization [79]. The rate of alloimmunization among transfusion-dependent thalassemia (TDT) patients is varying from 2.5–37% in different parts of the world [70, 87, 89]. The prevalence of anti-E, anti-c, and anti-c with anti-E in the Indian population is about 22–36%, 6.4%–38.8%, and 6.4%, respectively [90–92]. Relative immunogenicity of blood group antigen in a multi-transfused patient with an increase in a number of RBC unit exposure give the following grading: K > Jk^a > Lu^a > E > P1 > c > M > Le^b > C > Le^a > Fy^a > S [93]. Extended blood group antigen phenotyping should be done to reduce the risk of alloimmunization. Keeping that thing in mind; our blood center phenotyped 500 'O' grouped donors for 35 blood group antigens [94].

3.2.7 Adverse transfusion reactions

Patients dependent on blood transfusion for survival, are exposed to a variety of risks [71, 79]. Therefore, it is utmost important to improve blood safety, find ways to minimize or reduce transfusion requirements and less exposures to number of donors. The adverse transfusion events are:

- **Non-hemolytic febrile transfusion reactions:** This type of transfusion reactions was very common before the introduction of the leukoreduced red cell component and was reduced effectively by the use of this component. Patients who are prone to develop this type of reaction should be administered with antipyretics before their transfusions.

- **Allergic reactions**: Such reactions can progress from mild to severe mainly caused by the presence of IgE antibodies in plasma proteins. Recurrent allergic reactions can be markedly reduced by washing the red cells to remove the plasma. Patients with IgA deficiency and severe allergic reactions may require blood from IgA deficient donors.

- **Acute hemolytic reactions:** It's very unusual and the most common type arises due to errors in patient or donor identification in typing and compatibility testing. It is common to those thalassemia patients who take blood units from different blood centers. A blood center that strictly follows the WHO protocol for screening antibodies and full cross-match of donor unit, can avoid hemolytic reactions in patients.

- **Autoimmune hemolytic anemia:** One of the serious complications of blood transfusion that is commonly combined with alloimmunization. Sometimes compatible red cells may have short survival and hemoglobin may fall well below the pretransfusion level. To clinically manage this fatal reaction, steroids, immunosuppressive drugs and intravenous immunoglobulin should be administered, although benefits are fewer. If a patient undergoes a massive transfusions later in life may have such transfusion reaction frequently [95].

- **Delayed transfusion reactions:** These occur 5 to 10 days after transfusion and are characterized by anemia, malaise, and jaundice. These reactions may be due to an alloantibody that was not detectable at the time of transfusion or to the development of a new antibody. A sample should be sent to the Blood center to look for a new antibody and to re-crossmatch the last administered units.

- **Transfusion-related acute lung injury (TRALI):** Potentially severe complications normally caused by specific anti-neutrophil or anti-HAL antibodies that activate patients' neutrophil. It may sometimes occur due to the accumulation of the pro-inflammatory mediators during the storage of donor red cell [96, 97]. Management includes oxygen, administration of steroids and diuretics, and, when needed, assisted ventilation.

- **Transfusion-induced graft versus host disease (TI-GVHD):** caused by the viable lymphocytes in the donor's red cell unit, a rare but fatal complication due to transfusion. TI-GVHD may occur in immunosuppressed as well as immunocompetent patients. To avoid this, a blood transfusion of the family member's donated blood should be given after irradiation. Leucodepletion alone is inadequate for the prevention of this complication.

3.2.8 Transfusion transmitted infections (TTIs)

Blood safety depends on both donor health screening and donation testing. The strategy employed for a given infectious agent depends on the epidemiology of the particular agent in a given donor population, blood processing steps that might reduce transmission (such as pre-storage universal leucoreduction), and the availability of testing equipment and kits adapted for donor screening [98].

The different testing platforms can be used for screening TTIs. Tests that detect viral nucleic acid (NAT testing), a viral component (Hepatitis B surface antigen, or HBsAg; the p24 antigen of HIV), or the host's immune response to the infection (antibody testing performed using Enzyme linked immunosorbent assay (ELISA) or enzyme immunoassay (EIA)/chemiluminescence assay (CLIA) for antibodies such as anti-HIV, and anti-HBV). Any unit tested positive once for TTI must not be used for transfusion. Window period infections can be missed by ELSIA and chemiluminescence assay [98].

In general, window periods are shortest for NAT testing, longer for antigen testing, and longest for antibody detection. The lag time for anti-HIV to detect HIV infection can be as long as 21 days, for HBsAg test to detect HBV infection as long as 42 days, and for anti-HCV to detect HCV infection as long as 60 days. This lag period gets truncated (shortened) by direct tests for viral gene amplification with NAT [98]. Being costlier investigation than ELISA and chemiluminescence assay, NAT testing is still not available at many centers in developing countries like India [99].

Single unit NAT testing is more sensitive than using mini pool NAT where small numbers of donor samples are pooled [100]. Using this mini pool NAT of 10 samples, at our centre more than 8000 seronegative units were tested, out of those 44 donors were found positive for HBV, 5 for HIV and 2 for HCV. So ultimately these NAT positive units were stopped to be transfused to the patients [101]. Thalassemia and Sickle cell anemia patients should be transfused to the NAT tested unit [28]. In India only a few blood center hospital-based or private are doing either ID-NAT or mini-pooled NAT [99, 102–104]. In the year 2019 at our centre, as a part of the regular protocol, we tested 196 thalassemia major patients who are taking blood units from our centre only for transfusion, by ELISA and NAT (ID-NAT) for HIV1, HBV and HCV, the prevalence of HCV infection was found high by both the methods [105].

The testing algorithms for TTI s are also variable as per the testing facilities available at the blood centers. In the urban areas, screening for TTI is carried out by the ELISA technique with good quality measures while the remote rural areas are still left with a rapid test of questionable sensitivity. Moreover, in the remote rears where laboratory testing for TTI's is not quality assured, equipment is not calibrated and maintained, and the validation of results is not carried out. Even at the good centers that are doing ELISA using 3rd generation kits; not able to cut down the window period which can be achieved by 4th generation ELSIA. It's a big pressure on the Indian Blood center to adopt NAT for screening TTIs as Blood centers around the countries like USA, Canada, Australia, New Zealand, South Africa, and some countries in Europe and Asia have already used the same [106].

Because of the need for sensitivity in testing systems, TTI screening may lead to false biological false positive results. Many TTI test systems rely on cut-off values to determine whether a result is reactive or not, so the test results that fall close to a range of uncertainty may give the intermediate result. For such kind of indecisive results, extreme care needs to be taken with follow-up action for that particular donor, including confirmatory testing on the donation. The confirmed reactivity to certain TTIs such as HIV, HBV and HCV leads to permanent exclusion of the donor, whereas the risk of other TTIs such as malaria may have specified time deferrals [98].

3.2.9 Iron chelation and chelation

On an average, each unit of packed cells contains 200 to 250 mg of iron [28, 79]. A patient, who receives 15–30 units of pRBC units per year, receives an excess of 3–6 grams of elemental iron that results in to iron overload, a serious problem in massively transfused patients. Iron supplements are contraindicated as iron absorption may increase up to 1–2 gm. Serum ferritin, MRI of Liver and heart, and Liver biopsy would be good parameters to check the severity of iron over load in multitransfused patients. Iron chelation therapy should be started in patients whose serum ferritin value is >1000 μg/L after 10–15 transfusion. Different chelating agents are mentioned in the guidelines issued by the Ministry of Health & Family Welfare, India in 2016 for the prevention of hemoglobinopathies. They are Desferrioxamine (recommended dose is 25 mg-50 mg/kg/day) [71], Deferiprone (standard dose is 50 mg–100 mg/kg/day), Deferasirox (administered at a dose of 20 mg–40 mg/kg/day) and combination of desferrioxamine and deferiprone should be available for the patients. Before administering any chelating agent to the patient, the toxicity of an agent and required monitoring measures should be taken in account.

3.2.10 Molecular genotyping

Over a century, for detection of RBC antigen, a gold standard method, hemagglutination has been used to predict phenotype. Hemagglutination also term as serology is a sensitive, easy to perform, low costing and specific technique for the determination of RBC phenotype and is considered as optimal method for patient care. The serology technique reduces issuing time for blood units by extensive typing of donor's antigens. On other hand, with advances in immunohematology gives an understanding of the molecular basis of many blood group antigens. Molecular genotyping will help to type donors for a wider spectrum of minor blood group antigens and also genotype blood group antigens of multiply transfused patients such as sickle cell anemia or β-thalassemia or patients having positive direct antiglobulin test [106].

In multitransfused patients, haemagglutination fails to phenotype the patient's antigens due to donor-derived erythrocytes from previous transfusions. The molecular background of blood group polymorphisms is used for blood group antigen typing [107]. Previous studies have shown that molecular methods prove successful in determining the correct antigen profile of a multitransfused patient [108–110]. Both the blood donors and recipients can be genetically typed for all the clinically significant blood group antigens and antigen-matched blood can be provided to the recipient [108–112].

This approach could significantly reduce the rate of alloimmunization. Many PCR-based molecular detection assays are available. As per the laboratory facilities low throughput, medium- throughput and high-throughput PCR-based assays are available for blood group genotyping, PCR-RFLP technique though to be the first to be used for the purpose [107, 113, 114]. Many researchers around the world have used different PCR-based platform to genotype clinically significant antigens among multitransfused patients as well as in blood donors [115–123]. Our blood center has also typed regular voluntary blood donors, multitransfused patients (Thalassemia major & Sickle cell disease) and the tribal population [124, 125] for Rh, Kell, Duffy and Kidd blood group system; there was the statistically significant difference was observed in the phenotypic and genotypic prevalence of all these system's antigens especially in the thalassemia major patients.

4. Conclusion and future recommendations

Haemoglobinopathies in India are always the burning problem especially Beta-thalassemia major and Sickle cell disease; due to various aspects including screening of the patients in remote areas, lack of awareness about the severity of the diseases in rural as well as in urban areas, consanguine marriages, poor antenatal and prenatal screening tests, delay in timely detection of the diseased child, having misconceptions, myths, rigidity and superstitions among the general population, inert-caste marriages likewise many more adding to the burden.

SRKRC being the first charitable blood Centre in Surat city is providing safe blood for the last 44 years by following all the National guidelines. Just like what a blood centre should do, SRKRC is continuously updated with the current trends in transfusion medicine for the management of, especially multi transfused patients like Beta-thalassemia major and SCD. Starting from supplying perfectly crossed matched washed red cells or leuco-depleted pRBC's units to these patients. SRKRC has also implemented regular time interval strategies for irregular antibody screening, investigations TTI's, and providing the iron chelation therapy as well for batter management of these patients. Although for TTI's, ELISA is the mandatory test, in addition to that SRKRC is doing NAT testing which reduces the window period of TTI's and adds an extra layer of safety to the transfused blood units. Transfusion reactions are also one of the problems with these patients, antigen matched blood or antigen-negative blood (in case of alloantibody in-patient) should be transfused by typing patient and donor thoroughly with gold standard serology and advanced molecular genotyping techniques. SRKRC has developed a molecular genotyping facility for clinically significant blood group antigens that would serve the same purpose. As a blood centre, SRKRC is doing all above-mentioned possible transfusion practices and protocols that may help to enhance the time interval between two transfusions.

Along with routine blood centre activity, SRKRC is also running prevention and control programs for Beta-thalassemia and Sickle cell anemia for the last 16 years. This program includes the screening of the premarital, antenatal, PND and neonatal cases with proper counseling for every target population that significantly helps to prevent and control the disease.

Hence, it is suggested that nationalized policies are needed to be implemented at the micro-level for screening, counseling, prevention, blood transfusion and management of such patients to achieve the final goal of 'HAEMOGLOBINOPATHIES FREE COUNTRY'. India has many international, national and state-wise prevention and control programs for different diseases like HIV, Tuberculosis (TB), Malaria, SCD, etc., that include testing, medication and management of the individual patient at very cost-effective or free of cost manner. Likewise, for not just Beta-thalassemia but also for transfusion-dependent and severe hemoglobinopathies, nationalized prevention and control programs should be formed by combining the screening, counseling, blood transfusion and treatment aspects.

National Medical Commission (NMC) of India is running a doctor of medicine (MD) PG programme on the subject of Transfusion Medicine (TM) in most medical colleges in India. It is a clinical MD degree after MBBS and recognized by NMC and the curriculum completely covered all the advanced and clinical aspects related to Immune hematology, Blood Transfusion therapy, Blood Centre Direction, haemoglobinopathies and its management. More than 150 TM specialist doctors passing out every year in India, so enough specialist doctors would be available to meet the requirement of the concept programme. A concept, "District Haemoglobinopathy Clinic" along with Regional Blood Centre, programme under the name of #Make Country Free from Haemoglobinopathies is to be recommended.

Aim, Facilities and goals of the "District Haemoglobinopathy Clinic" should be like;

4.1 Diagnosis, Registry and Management of diagnosed patients

- Generation of 'Nationalized unique ID' and 'National haemoglobinopathy Registry' suffering from haemoglobinopathy in a particular district.

- Regional Blood Centre: As described above, under TM specialist directions advanced fully equipped blood centre establishment at the district level for the high quality and safest blood products provision to all diagnosed patients. District regional blood centre should have quality and audit responsibility of all other blood centres where pt's is taking blood. Moreover, test discrepancies and complicated patients should be referred to the district clinic for further investigation and quality care therapy.

- Transfusion Centre: Under the TM specialist, a transfusion centre should be established for monitoring of serum ferritin and iron for starting chelation therapy, and assured blood unit for the transfusion. In addition, under the unique ID, patient's record of each transfusion, treatment and testing should be maintained in Web software linked and visible to all care giving physicians, which would be helpful in-patient management if he/she will migrate from one place to the other.

4.2 Watertight screening, counseling and prevention for diseases

- Goal of Zero marriage between two carrier persons: Screening for all hemoglobinopathy with HPLC of premarital/adolescent age of the all-high-risk group people of districts, counseling and prevention to achieve Goal of Zero marriage in between two haemoglobinopathy disease carrier persons in a particular district.

- Goal of Zero conception of the foetus with the homozygous state: Screening for all hemoglobinopathy with HPLC of all married couples of the all-high-risk group people of districts, counseling and prevention to achieve Goal of Zero conception of the foetus with the homozygous state in particular district couples who missed at pre-marital/adolescent stage.

- Goal of 100% Newborn screening for haemoglobinopathies: Screening for all hemoglobinopathy with HPLC of all newborns of the districts to achieve Goal of 100% Newborn screening for haemoglobinopathies in a particular district and to enroll start the early quality care & medical treatment for the diagnosed newborn at District haemoglobinopathy clinic.

- 100% mandatory hemoglobinopathies screening report at pre-marital/adolescent age stage during the education and before marriage registration of couples, identifying the carrier state person, counseling and prevention for the same.

All these facilities at one place would be a great help to an affected child and a family that they should not have to roam here and there, although to set up such facilities Government aids are much needed.

These district-level clinics should be integrated inter-districts through Nodal officers to create State-level registry and database; these State-level reference clinics should be integrated Inter-State through Zone level officer of the Country to create National level registry and all databases. These could be assessable by caregiving physicians anywhere in the country, with all history and given therapeutic management, which could be helpful for better prospective care and increase the quality of life of patients. Only by implementing this level of concept programme, we could make Country Free from Haemoglobinopathies and zero birth of hemoglobinopathy case can be achieved in the Country.

Author details

Avani Shah, Sumit Bharadva*, Parizad Patel and Kanchan Mishra
Surat Raktadan Kendra and Research Centre, Surat, Gujarat, India

*Address all correspondence to: sumit_bharadva@hotmail.com

References

[1] Polus RK. Prevalence of hemoglobinopathies among marrying couples in Erbil province of Iraq. Iraqi Journal of Hematology. 2017;**6**(2):90

[2] Wheatherall D, Clegg J. The Thalassemia Syndromes. Oxford: England: Blackwell Science Ltd; 2001

[3] Khan K, Zahoor S. Pattern of Hemoglobinopathies on HPLC among patients referred to selected centers in Peshawar, Pakistan. Rawal Medical Journal. 2018;**43**(4):623-626

[4] Williams TN, Weatherall DJ. World distribution, population genetics, and health burden of the hemoglobinopathies. Cold Spring Harbor perspectives in medicine. 2012;**2**(9):a011692

[5] Goonasekera HW, Paththinige CS, Dissanayake VH. Population screening for hemoglobinopathies. Annual Review of Genomics and Human Genetics. 2018;**19**:355-380

[6] Cao A, Kan YW. The prevention of thalassemia. Cold Spring Harbor perspectives in medicine. 2013;**3**(2): a011775

[7] Madan N, Sharma S, Sood SK, Colah R, Bhatia HM. Frequency of β-thalassemia trait and other hemoglobinopathies in northern and Western India. Indian Journal of Human Genetics. 2010;**16**(1):16

[8] Sengupta M. Thalassemia among the tribal communities of India. Internet Journal of Biological Anthropology. 2008;**1**(2):1-9

[9] Verma IC, Saxena R, Kohli S. Past, present & future scenario of thalassaemic care & control in India. The Indian Journal of Medical Research. 2011;**134**(4):507

[10] Christianson A, Howson CP, Modell B. March of Dimes: Global report on birth defects, the hidden toll of dying and disabled children. White Plains, New York: March of Dimes Birth Defects Foundation; 2005

[11] Bremner J, Frost A, Haub C, Mather M, Ringheim K, Zuehlke E. World population highlights: Key findings from PRB's 2010 world population data sheet. Population Bulletin. 2010;**65**(2):1-2

[12] Grow K, Vashist M, Abrol P, Sharma S, Yadav R. Beta thalassemia in India: current status and the challenges ahead. International Journal of Pharmacy and Pharmaceutical Sciences. 2014;**6**(4):28-33

[13] Marwaha N. Whole blood and component use in resource poor settings. Biologicals. 2010;**38**(1):68-71

[14] Anand, Kumar K, Radhakrishna N, Sachdeva A. Management of thalassemia in Indian perspective. Thalassemia: National Guidelines for management of transfusion-dependent thalassemia and non-transfusion dependent thalassemia; Thalassemia International Foundation, Cyprus; 2014. pp. 296-302

[15] Modell B, Petrou M. The problem of the hemoglobinopathies in India. Indian Journal of Hematology. 1983;**1**:5-16

[16] Gorakshakar AC, Colah RB. Cascade screening for β-thalassemia: A practical approach for identifying and counseling carriers in India. Indian Journal of Community Medicine. 2009;**34**(4):354

[17] Bhatia HM, Shanbagh SR, Baxi AJ, Bapat JP, Sharma RS. Genetic studies among the endogamous groups of Lohanas of North and West India. Human heredity. 1976;**26**(4):298-305

[18] Mukherjee MB, Gangakhedkar RR, Sathe MS. Abnormal hemoglobin, G6PD deficiency and their pattern of

interaction in the tribal population of Valsad district (Gujarat). Indian J Hematol Blood Transf. 1993;**11**:227-231

[19] Rao VR. Genetic atlas of the Indian tribes. Institute of Immunohaematology. Mumbai: Indian Council of Medical Research; 1986

[20] Patel AG, Shah AP, Sorathiya SM, Gupte SC. Hemoglobinopathies in South Gujarat population and incidence of anemia in them. Indian journal of human genetics. 2012;**18**(3):294

[21] Ryan K, Bain B, Worthington D, James J, Plews D, Mason A, et al. Significant haemoglobinopathies: Guidelines for screening and diagnosis. British Journal of Haematology. 2010;**149**(1):35-49

[22] Alswaidi FM, O'brien SJ. Premarital screening programmes for haemoglobinopathies, HIV and hepatitis viruses: Review and factors affecting their success. Journal of medical screening. 2009;**16**(1):22-28

[23] Bain BJ. Haemoglobinopathy diagnosis: Algorithms, lessons and pitfalls. Blood Reviews. 2011;**25**(5):205-213

[24] Lewis SM, Bain BJ, Bates I, Dacie JV. Dacie and Lewis practical haematology. UK: Churchill Livingstone; 2006

[25] Mohanty D, Colah R. Eds Laboratory Manual for Screening, Diagnosis and Molecular analysis in Hemoglobinopathies and Red Cell Enzymopathies. 1st ed. Mumbai: Bhalani Publishing House; 2008

[26] Ghosh K, Colah R, Manglani M, Choudhry VP, Verma I, Madan N, et al. Guidelines for screening, diagnosis and management of hemoglobinopathies. Indian Journal of Human Genetics. 2014;**20**(2):101

[27] U.S. Health and Human Services, Centers for Disease Control and Prevention. Hemoglobinopathies. In: Current practices for screening, confirmation and follow-up. Association of Public Health Laboratories, US; 2015

[28] National Health Mission Guidelines on Hemoglobinopathies in India Prevention and control of hemoglobinopathies in India-Thalassemia. Sickle cell disease and other variant hemoglobins. Delhi: Ministry of Health and Family Welfare, Govt of India; 2016

[29] Mathews V. Allogeneic stem cell transplantation for thalassemia major. Regenerative Medicine: Laboratory to Clinic. Switzerland: Springer; 2017. pp. 343-357

[30] Srivastava JK, Sinha N, Behera SK, Panja S, Sarkar BN, Rao VR. Knowledge, attitude and practice study of beta-thalassemia in rural Bengal. Genetics Clinic. 2011;**4**(4):13-15

[31] Chawla S, Singh RK, Lakkakula BV, Vadlamudi RR. Attitudes and beliefs among high-and low-risk population groups towards β-thalassemia prevention: a cross-sectional descriptive study from India. Journal of community genetics. 2017;**8**(3):159-166

[32] Chandy M. Developing a national thalassemia control programme for India. In: Ghosh K, Colah R, editors. Control and management of thalassemia and other hemoglobinopathies in the indian subcontinent-synoptic views. Mumbai: National Institute of Immunohaematology; 2008

[33] Warghade S, Britto J, Haryan R, Dalvi T, Bendre R, Chheda P, et al. Prevalence of hemoglobin variants and hemoglobinopathies using cation-exchange high-performance liquid chromatography in central reference laboratory of India: A report of 65779 cases. Journal of laboratory physicians. 2018 Jan;**10**(01):073-079

[34] Rao VR, Gorakshakar AC. Sickle cell hemoglobin, beta-thalassemia and G6PD deficiency in tribes of Maharashtra, India. Gene geography: A computerized bulletin on human gene frequencies. 1990;**4**(3):131-134

[35] Balgir RS. Genetic heterogeneity of population structure in 15 major scheduled tribes in central-eastern India: A study of immuno-hematological disorders. Indian Journal of Human Genetics. 2006;**12**(2):86-92

[36] Chatterjee N, Mishra A, Soni R, Kulkarni H, Mamtani M, Shrivasatava M. Bayesian estimates of the prevalence of β-thalassemia trait in voluntary blood donors of central India: a survey. Hemoglobin. 2010;**34**(6):548-560

[37] Munkongdee T, Chen P, Winichagoon P, Fucharoen S, Paiboonsukwong K. Update in laboratory diagnosis of thalassemia. Frontiers in Molecular Biosciences. 2020;7:74

[38] Hendrix MM, Cuthbert CD, Cordovado SK. Assessing the performance of Dried-Blood-Spot DNA extraction methods in next generation sequencing. International Journal of Neonatal Screening. 2020;**6**(2):36

[39] Mifflin TE. Setting Up a PCR Laboratory. In: Dieffenbach CW, Dveksler GS, editors. PCR Primer: a Laboratory Manual. 2nd ed. Cold Spring Harbor, NY: Cold Spring Harbor Laboratory Press; 2003. pp. 5-14

[40] Mishra KK, Patel P, Bhukhanvala DS, Shah A, Ghosh K. A multiplex ARMS PCR approach to detection of common β-globin gene mutations. Analytical Biochemistry. 2017;**537**:93-98

[41] Bhukhanvala DS, Italia K, Sawant P, Colah R, Ghosh K, Gupte SC. Molecular characterization of β-thalassemia in four communities in South Gujarat—codon 30 (G→ A) a predominant mutation in the Kachhiya Patel community. Annals of hematology. 2013;**92**(11):1473-1476

[42] Varawalla NY, Old JM, Sarkar R, Venkatesan R, Weatherall DJ. The spectrum of β-thalassaemia mutations on the Indian subcontinent: The basis for prenatal diagnosis. British Journal of Haematology. 1991;**78**(2):242-247

[43] Mukherjee MB, Lu CY, Ducrocq R, Gangakhedkar RR, Colah RB, Kadam MD, et al. Effect of α-thalassemia on sickle-cell anemia linked to the Arab-Indian haplotype in India. American Journal of Hematology. 1997;**55**(2):104-109

[44] Iyer SR, Iyer RR, Oza GD, Rane RM, Khandwala RM, Desai PK, et al. Sickle cell syndromes in and around Bardoli. The Journal of the Association of Physicians of India. 1994;**42**(11):885-887

[45] Newton CR, Graham A, Heptinstall LE, Powell SJ, Summers C, Kalsheker N, et al. Analysis of any point mutation in DNA. The amplification refractory mutation system (ARMS). Nucleic Acids Research. 1989;**17**(7):2503-2516

[46] Ristaldi MS, Pirastu M, Rosatelli C, Monni G, Erlich H, Saiki R, et al. Prenatal diagnosis of β-thalassaemia in Mediterranean populations by dot blot analysis with DNA amplification and allele specific oligonucleotide probes. Prenatal Diagnosis. 1989;**9**(9):629-638

[47] Bhardwaj U, Zhang YH, McCabe ER. Neonatal hemoglobinopathy screening: molecular genetic technologies. Molecular Genetics and Metabolism. 2003;**80**(1-2):129-137

[48] Joshi VA, Mancini-DiNardo D, Funke BH. Selection of a platform for mutation detection. Current protocols in human genetics. 2008;**56**(1):7-15

[49] He J, Song W, Yang J, Lu S, Yuan Y, Guo J, et al. Next-generation sequencing

improves thalassemia carrier screening among premarital adults in a high prevalence population: the Dai nationality. China. Genetics in Medicine. 2017 Sep;**19**(9):1022-1031

[50] Shang X, Peng Z, Ye Y, Zhang X, Chen Y, Zhu B, et al. Rapid targeted next-generation sequencing platform for molecular screening and clinical genotyping in subjects with hemoglobinopathies. eBioMedicine. 2017;**23**:150-159

[51] Huang Q, Liu Z, Liao Y, Chen X, Zhang Y, Li Q. Multiplex fluorescence melting curve analysis for mutation detection with dual-labeled, self-quenched probes. PLoS One. 2011;**6**(4): e19206

[52] Xiong F, Huang Q, Chen X, Zhou Y, Zhang X, Cai R, et al. A melting curve analysis–based PCR assay for one-step genotyping of β-thalassemia mutations: a multicenter validation. The Journal of Molecular Diagnostics. 2011;**13**(4): 427-435

[53] Sirichotiyakul S, Saetung R, Sanguansermsri T. Analysis of β-thalassemia mutations in northern Thailand using an automated fluorescence DNA sequencing technique. Hemoglobin. 2003;**27**(2): 89-95

[54] Korf BR, Rehm HL. New approaches to molecular diagnosis. Journal of the American Medical Association. 2013;**309**(14):1511-1521

[55] Schouten JP, McElgunn CJ, Waaijer R, Zwijnenburg D, Diepvens F, Pals G. Relative quantification of 40 nucleic acid sequences by multiplex ligation-dependent probe amplification. Nucleic Acids Research. 2002;**30**(12):e57

[56] Zhang H, Li C, Li J, Hou S, Chen D, Yan H, et al. Next-generation sequencing improves molecular epidemiological characterization of thalassemia in Chenzhou region, PR China. Journal of Clinical Laboratory Analysis. 2019;**33**(4):e22845

[57] Colah R, Italia K, Gorakshakar A. Burden of thalassemia in India: The road map for control. Pediatric Hematology Oncology Journal. 2017;**2**(4):79-84

[58] Sharma A. Thalassemia patients require centralised blood transfusion [Internet]. Express Healthcare, India. 2021 [cited 2021 July 18]. Available from: https://www.expresshealthcare.in/news/thalassemia-patients-require-centralised-blood transfusion/429595/

[59] Shah FT, Sayani F, Trompeter S, Drasar E, Piga A. Challenges of blood transfusions in β-thalassemia. Blood Reviews. 2019;**37**:100588.-70

[60] Sirchia G, Zanella A, Parravicini A, Rebulla P, Morelati F, Masera G. Red cell alloantibodies in thalassemia major: results of an Italian cooperative study. Transfusion. 1985;**25**(2):110-2-110-11071

[61] Thompson AA, Cunningham MJ, Singer ST, Neufeld EJ, Vichinsky E, Yamashita R, et al. Thalassemia Clinical Research Network Investigators. Red cell alloimmunization in a diverse population of transfused patients with thalassaemia. British Journal of Haematology. 2011;**153**(1):121-128

[62] Thuret I, Pondarré C, Loundou A, Steschenko D, Girot R, Bachir D, et al. Complications and treatment of patients with β-thalassemia in France: results of the National Registry. Haematologica. 2010;**95**(5):724

[63] World Health Organization. Haemoglobin concentrations for the diagnosis of anaemia and assessment of severity. Geneva: World Health Organization; 2011

[64] Carson JL, Stanworth SJ, Roubinian N, Fergusson DA, Triulzi D, Doree C, et al. Transfusion thresholds

and other strategies for guiding allogeneic red blood cell transfusion. Cochrane database of systematic reviews. 2016;**10**:1-93

[65] Carson JL, Guyatt G, Heddle NM, Grossman BJ, Cohn CS, Fung MK, et al. Clinical practice guidelines from the AABB: red blood cell transfusion thresholds and storage. Journal of the American Medical Association. 2016;**316**(19):2025-2035

[66] Eleftheriou A. Thalassemia International Federation: Guidelines for the clinical management of thalassemia. Thalassemia International Federation Nicosia Cyprus. 2008

[67] Taher A, Vichinsky E, Musallam K, Cappellini MD, Viprakasit V. Guidelines for the management of non-transfusion dependent thalassaemia (NTDT). Thalassemia International Federation, Nicosia Cyprus. 2014

[68] United Kingdom Thalassaemia Society. Standards for the clinical care of children and adults with thalassaemia in the UK. 3rd ed. UK: UK Thalassemia Society; 2016

[69] Standards of care guidelines for thalassemia. Children's Hospital & Research Center Oakland. California, US. 2012

[70] Sayani F, Warner M, Wu J, Wong-Rieger D, Humphreys K, Odame I. Guidelines for the clinical care of patients with thalassemia in Canada. ON, Canada: Anemia Institute for Research & Education, Thalassemia Foundation of Canada; 2009

[71] Rao GH, Eastlund T, Jagannathan L. Handbook of Blood Banking and 7. Transfusion Medicine. In: Pathare AV, editor. Transfusion Therapy for Hemoglobinopathies, Handbook of Blood Banking and Transfusion Medicine. India: JP Medical Publishers; 2005. pp. 173-185

[72] Brittenham GM, Griffith PM, Nienhuis AW, McLaren CE, Young NS, Tucker EE, et al. Efficacy of deferoxamine in preventing complications of iron overload in patients with thalassemia major. New England Journal of Medicine. 1994;**331**(9):567-573

[73] Olivieri NF, Brittenham GM, Matsui D, Berkovitch M, Blendis LM, Cameron RG, et al. Iron-chelation therapy with oral deferiprone in patients with thalassemia major. New England Journal of Medicine. 1995;**332**(14): 918-922

[74] Cappellini N, Cohen A, Elefteriou A, Piga A, Porter J. TIF Guidelines for the clinical management of thalassemia. Cyprus: Thalassemia International Federation; 2000. pp. 9-14-9-85

[75] Tubman VN, Fung EB, Vogiatzi M, Thompson AA, Rogers ZR, Neufeld EJ, et al. Guidelines for the standard monitoring of patients with thalassemia: report of the thalassemia longitudinal cohort. Journal of pediatrichematology/ oncology. 2015;**37**(3):e162

[76] Azarkeivan A, Ansari S, Ahmadi MH, Hajibeigy B, Maghsudlu M, Nasizadeh S, et al. Blood transfusion and alloimmunization in patients with thalassemia: multicenter study. Pediatrichematology and Oncology. 2011;**28**(6):479-485

[77] Singer ST, Wu V, Mignacca R, Kuypers FA, Morel P, Vichinsky EP. Alloimmunization and erythrocyte autoimmunization in transfusion-dependent thalassemia patients of predominantly Asian descent Blood. The Journal of the American Society of Hematology. 2000;**96**(10):3369-3373

[78] Ameen R, Al-Shemmari S, Al-Humood S, Chowdhury RI, Al-Eyaadi O, Al-Bashir A. RBC alloimmunization and autoimmunization among transfusion-dependent Arab

thalassemia patients. Transfusion. 2003;**43**(11):1604-1610

[79] Cappellini MD, Cohen A, Porter J, Taher A, Viprakasit V. Guidelines for the management of transfusion dependent thalassaemia (TDT). Nicosia, Cyprus: Thalassaemia International Federation; 2014. p. 91

[80] Joshi SR, Shah Al-Bulushi SN, Ashraf T. Development of blood transfusion service in Sultanate of Oman. Asian J Transfus Sci. 2010;**4**:34-40

[81] Bharucha ZS, Jolly JG, Ghosh K. Standards for Blood Banks and Blood Transfusion Services. New Delhi: Ministry of Health and Family Welfare; 2007. pp. 83-4.-93

[82] Piomelli S, Seaman C, Reibman J, Tytun A, Graziano J, Tabachnik N, et al. Separation of younger red cells with improved survival in vivo: An approach to chronic transfusion therapy. Proceedings of the National Academy of Sciences. 1978;**75**(7):3474-3478

[83] Cohen AR, Schmidt JM, Martin MB, Barnsley W, Schwartz E. Clinical trial of young red cell transfusions. The Journal of pediatrics. 1984;**104**(6):865-868

[84] Simon TL, Sohmer P, Nelson EJ. Extended survival of neocytes produced by a new system. Transfusion. 1989;**29**(3):221-225

[85] Kevy SV, Jacobson MS, Fosburg M, Renaud M, Scanlon A, Carmen R, et al. A new approach to neocyte transfusion: Preliminary report. Journal of clinical apheresis. 1988;**4**(4):194-197

[86] Spanos T, Ladis V, Palamidou F, Papassotiriou I, Banagi A, Premetis E, et al. The impact of neocyte transfusion in the management of thalassaemia. Voxsanguinis. 1996;**70**(4):217-223

[87] Collins AF, Dias GC, Haddad S, Talbot R, Herst R, Tyler BJ, et al. Evaluation of a new neocyte transfusion preparation vs washed cell transfusion in patients with homozygous beta thalassemia. Transfusion. 1994;**34**:517

[88] Spanos TH, Karageorga M, Ladis V, Peristeri J, Hatziliami A, Kattamis C. Red cell alloantibodies in patients with thalassemia. Voxsanguinis. 1990;**58**(1): 50-55

[89] Wang LY, Liang DC, Liu HC, Chang FC, Wang CL, Chan YS, et al. Alloimmunization among patients with transfusion-dependent thalassemia in Taiwan. Transfusion Medicine. 2006;**16**(3):200-203

[90] Zaman S, Chaurasia R, Chatterjee K, Thapliyal RM. Prevalence and specificity of RBC alloantibodies in Indian patients attending a tertiary care hospital. Advances in hematology. 2014;**1**:2014

[91] Thakral B, Saluja K, Sharma RR, Marwaha N. Red cell alloimmunization in a transfused patient population: A study from a tertiary care hospital in north India. Hematology. 2008;**13**(5):313-318

[92] Jariwala K, Mishra K, Ghosh K. Comparative study of alloimmunization against red cell antigens in sickle cell disease & thalassaemia major patients on regular red cell transfusion. The Indian journal of medical research. 2019;**149**(1):34

[93] Stack G, Tormey CA. Detection rate of blood group alloimmunization based on real-world testing practices and kinetics of antibody induction and evanescence. Transfusion. 2016;**56**(11): 2662-7-2662-266108

[94] Shah A, Jariwala K, Gupte S, Sharma P, Mishra K, Ghosh K. Pattern of distribution of 35 red cell antigens in regular voluntary blood donors of South Gujarat, India. Transfusion and Apheresis Science. 2018;**57**(5): 672-5-672-67109

[95] Rebulla P, Modell B. Transfusion requirements and effects in patients with thalassaemia major. The Lancet. 1991;**337**(8736):277-280

[96] Vlaar AP, Juffermans NP. Transfusion-related acute lung injury: A clinical review. The Lancet. 2013;**382**(9896):984-994

[97] Swanson K, Dwyre DM, Krochmal J, Raife TJ. Transfusion-related acute lung injury (TRALI): Current clinical and pathophysiologic considerations. Lung. 2006;**184**(3):177-185

[98] Roman L, Armstrong B, Smart E. Reviewer for Second Edition: So-Yong Kwon. Donation testing and transfusion transmissible infections. Vol. 15. ISBT Science Series, Netherland; 2020. pp. 192-206-192-113

[99] Ghosh K, Mishra K. Nucleic acid amplification testing in Indian blood banks: A review with perspectives. Indian Journal of Pathology and Microbiology. 2017;**60**(3):313

[100] Ghosh K, Mishra KK, Trivedi A, Sosa S, Patel K. Assessment of semi-automated nucleic acid testing programme in a Regional Blood Transfusion Centre. British Journal of Biomedical Science. 2017;**74**(1): 42-7-42-4115

[101] Mishra KK, Trivedi A, Sosa S, Patel K, Ghosh K. NAT positivity in seronegative voluntary blood donors from western India. Transfusion and Apheresis Science. 2017;**56**(2): 175-8-175-17116

[102] Makroo RN, Choudhury N, Jagannathan L, Parihar-Malhotra M, Raina V, Chaudhary RK, et al. Multicenter evaluation of individual donor nucleic acid testing (NAT) for simultaneous detection of human immunodeficiency virus-1 & hepatitis B & C viruses in Indian blood donors. Indian Journal of Medical Research. 2008;**127**(2):117

[103] Naidu NK, Bharucha ZS, Sonawane V, Ahmed I. Nucleic acid testing: Is it the only answer for safe Blood in India? Asian Journal of Transfusion Science. 2016;**10, 1**:79-118

[104] Pathak S, Chakraborty T, Singh S, Dubey R. Impact of PCR-based Multiplex Minipool NAT on Donor Blood Screening at a Tertiary Care Hospital Blood Bank in North India. International Journal. 2021;**4**(1):570-119

[105] Mishra K, Shah A, Patel K, Ghosh K, Bharadva S. Seroprevalence of HBV, HCV and HIV-1 and correlation with molecular markers among multi-transfused thalassemia patients in Western India. Mediterranean Journal of Hematology and Infectious Diseases. 2020;**12**(1):120

[106] Quirino MG, Colli CM, Macedo LC, Sell AM, Visentainer JE. Methods for blood group antigens detection: cost-effectiveness analysis of phenotyping and genotyping. Hematology, Transfusion and Cell Therapy. 2019;41:44-9.-4121

[107] Avent ND. Large-scale blood group genotyping–clinical implications. British Journal of Haematology. 2009;**144**(1):3-13

[108] Guelsin GA, Sell AM, Castilho L, Masaki VL, Melo FC, Hashimoto MN, et al. Benefits of blood group genotyping in multi-transfused patients from the south of Brazil. Journal of Clinical Laboratory Analysis. 2010;**24**(5):311-316

[109] Hojjati MT, Einollahi N, Nabatchian F, Pourfathollah AA, Mahdavi MR. Allele-specific oligonucleotide polymerase chain reaction for the determination of Rh C/c and Rh E/e antigens in thalassaemic patients. Blood Transfusion. 2011;**9**(3):301

[110] Westhoff CM. The potential of blood group genotyping for transfusion medicine practice. Immunohematology. 2008;**24**(4):190-195

[111] Gorakshakar A, Gogri H, Ghosh K. Evolution of technology for molecular genotyping in blood group systems. The Indian Journal of Medical Research. 2017;**146**(3):305

[112] Reid ME, Rios M, Yazdanbakhsh K. Applications of molecular biology techniques to transfusion medicine. Semin Hematol. 2000;**37**(2):166-176

[113] Reid ME, Rios M, Powell VI, Charles-Pierre D, Malavade V. DNA from blood samples can be used to genotype patients who have recently received a transfusion. Transfusion. 2000;**40**(1):48-53

[114] Guelsin GA, Sell AM, Castilho L, Masaki VL, Melo FC, Hashimoto MN, et al. Genetic polymorphisms of Rh, Kell, Duffy and Kidd systems in a population from the State of Paraná, southern Brazil. Revistabrasileira de hematologia e hemoterapia. 2011;**33**:21-25

[115] Kulkarni S, Choudhary B, Gogri H, Patil S, Manglani M, Sharma R, et al. Molecular genotyping of clinically important blood group antigens in patients with thalassaemia. The Indian Journal of Medical Research. 2018;**148**(6):713-131

[116] Costa DC, Pellegrino J Jr, Guelsin GA, Ribeiro KA, Gilli SC, Castilho L. Molecular matching of red blood cells is superior to serological matching in sickle cell disease patients. Revistabrasileira de hematologia e hemoterapia. 2013;**35**:35-38

[117] Ye Z. Comparison of blood group molecular genotyping to traditional serological phenotyping in patients with chronic or recent blood transfusion. Journal of Biosciences and Medicines. 2016;**4**(03):1

[118] Osman NH, Sathar J, Leong CF, Zulkifli NF, Sabudin RZ, Othman A, et al. Importance of extended blood group genotyping in multiply transfused patients. Transfusion and Apheresis Science. 2017;**56**(3):410-6-410-41134

[119] MNS, Duffy, and Kell blood groups among the Uygur population of Xinjiang, China. Genetics and Molecular Research. 2017;**16**(1):1601-9176-1601-9135

[120] Nathalang O, Intharanut K, Siriphanthong K, Nathalang S, Kupatawintu P. Duffy blood group genotyping in Thai blood donors. Annals of Laboratory Medicine. 2015;**35**(6):618-23-618-618136

[121] Martins ML, da Silva AR, Santos HC, Alves MT, Schmidt LC, Vertchenko SB, et al. Duffy blood group system: New genotyping method and distribution in a Brazilian extra-Amazonian population. Molecular and Cellular Probes. 2017;**35**:20-6.137

[122] Flôres MA, Visentainer JE, Guelsin GA, de Souza FA, de Melo FC, Hashimoto MN, et al. Rh, Kell, Duffy, Kidd and Diego blood group system polymorphism in Brazilian Japanese descendants. Transfusion and Apheresis Science. 2014;**50**(1):123-8.13

[123] Xuereb K, Debono J, Borg JJ. Validation of a Polymerase Chain Reaction technique for Kidd blood group genotyping. Malta Journal of Health Sciences. 2015;**2**(2):66-69

[124] Shah A, Patel P, Patel K, Patel B, Jariwala K, Sharma P, et al. Comparison of serology and molecular detection of common red cell antigens in multitransfused thalassemia major and sickle cell disease patients. Transfusion and Apheresis Science. 2020;**59**(1):102599

[125] Shah A, Ghosh K, Sharma P, Mishra K. Phenotyping of Rh, Kell, Duffy and Kidd blood group antigens among non-tribal and tribal population of South Gujarat and its implication in preventing alloimmunization in multitransfused patients. Mediterranean Journal of Hematology and Infectious Diseases. 2018;**10**(1):1-4

Section 5

Maternal Hepatitis Infections

Chapter 6

Maternal Hepatitis Infections: Determining Seroprevalence of Hepatitis B and C Virus Infections and Associated Risk Factors among Healthy Mothers in Addis Ababa, Ethiopia

Habtamu Biazin Kebede and Seifegebriel Teshome

Abstract

Introduction: Viral hepatitis is a global public health problem affecting millions of people every year, causing disability and death. Hepatitis B (HBV) and hepatitis C (HCV) viruses spread horizontally, mainly through sexual contact and contaminated needles, and vertically. Both cause considerable morbidity and mortality worldwide. Maternal infection is a risk factor for vertical transmission. **Objective**: To determine the seroprevalence of HBsAg and anti-HCV antibody among non-pregnant, apparently healthy mothers and to identify potential risk factors associated with HBV or HCV infection. **Methods**: A community based cross sectional study was conducted on 454 apparently healthy women, in Addis Ababa, Ethiopia from May 2016 to June 2017. A systematic random sampling method was used to recruit participants. **Result**: A total of 454 mothers were enrolled. Seroprevalence of HBsAg and HCV was found to be 3.7% and 2.0%, respectively. HBc antibody was detected in 36.3% of the mothers. None of the participants was co-infected with both viruses. Previous history of liver disease, history of jaundice, HIV infection, and family history of liver disease were significantly associated with HBV infection. Marital status, caring for hepatitis patients, and a history of liver disease were factors significantly associated with HCV infection. **Conclusion**: Apparently, healthy mothers in Addis Ababa had intermediate level of endemicity for hepatitis B and C infections Routine screening and vaccination of high-risk reproductive mothers against HBV is advisable. Emphasis should be given to health education and promotion of infection control practices. Population based studies are strongly recommended to help monitor disease transmission patterns and to design evidence-based interventions against the spread of hepatitis infections in Ethiopia.

Keywords: Sero-prevalence, risk factors, hepatitis B and C virus, apparently healthy mothers

1. Introduction

Viral hepatitis is one of the major causes of chronic liver disease and liver failure. In many countries, viral hepatitis is the leading cause of liver transplants. Such end-stage treatments are expensive, easily reaching up to hundreds of thousands of dollars per person [1]. In addition, viral hepatitis places a heavy burden on the economy of nations due to loss of productivity. Although the burden of viral hepatitis is very high, it has not received the attention it deserved from the global community [1, 2]. Various reasons account for this negligence, including the relatively recent discovery of the causative viruses, the mostly silent or benign nature of the disease in its early stages, and the insidious way in which it causes chronic liver disease [1].

Among viral hepatitis, hepatitis B and C infections are more often seen in blood, tissue, or organ recipients and people working or receiving treatment in health care facilities [2]. The WHO has estimated that there are more than 2 billion people infected with hepatitis B virus (HBV) and about 378 million HBV carriers worldwide, leading to approximately 620, 000 HBV related deaths every year [2, 3]. Further, it has been reported that 4.5 million new HBV infections occur worldwide each year, of which a quarter progresses to liver disease [2, 3].

HBV infection is endemic in Asia and sub-Saharan Africa thought to be the main etiological factor in over 75% of the chronic liver disease burden [3]. In sub-Saharan Africa, the prevalence of HBV surface antigen (HBsAg), which indicates active infection, is 3–20% and prevalence of markers for past exposure range from 60 to 99.Since Ethiopia is located in Sub-Saharan Africa, it is considered an area of high endemicity for HBV infection.

Meanwhile, approximately 170 million individuals are infected with hepatitis C virus worldwide, leading to approximately 250 000 to 350 000 deaths per year [4].

Viral hepatitis is a key public health problem that poses an enormous risk for disease transmission in the general population, especially in children and mothers [2]. Reliable epidemiological data are essential for planning health programs and identifying risk groups, For example, the selection of appropriate treatment depends on the genotype of the virus, the presence or absence of cirrhosis, and on the degree of liver fibrosis [2]. Therefore, it is important to know the number of people infected with and dying from hepatitis related liver disease, the prevalence of hepatitis related morbidity, and the distribution of genotypes and fibrosis stages [3]. Unfortunately, estimates of these key epidemiological parameters are limited by the lack of data from in developing countries like Ethiopia.

In Ethiopia, only few community-based seroepidemiology studies have previously been done on the prevalence of HBV and HCV. These studies, which were investigating the prevalence of these viruses among pregnant mothers, blood donors, HIV infected individuals, health care workers, and medical waste handlers, have indicated that hepatitis infections are endemic in Ethiopia, with varying levels of endemicity from region to region [5]. However, community based hepatitis studies focusing on the prevalence of hepatitis B or/and C infection in mothers have not been conducted. Thus, the current study aims to measure the prevalence of hepatitis B and C infection and contributing factors among apparently healthy mothers. This study is important to define the prevalence of these viral infections and associated risks among apparently healthy mothers, in order to adopt effective preventive strategies, guidelines, and educational programmers. Overall, screening asymptomatic people is important for early diagnosis and intervention.

2. Methods and materials

2.1 Study area

This study was conducted in Addis Ababa city, which has a population of about 3.6 million and an average household size of 5.8 persons per household [6].

According to the 2007 national census, 98.6% of the housing units in Addis Ababa have access to safe drinking water. In addition, 14.9% have flush toilets, 70.7% have pit toilet, and 14.3% have no toilet facilities [7]. Values for other reported common indicators of the standard of living for Addis Ababa showed that as of 2012 0.1% of the inhabitants fall into the lowest wealth quintile [6]. Adult literacy for men and woman is 93.6% and 79.9% respectively the highest in the nation for both sexes. Further, the civic (urban) infant mortality rate is 45 infant deaths per 1,000 live births, which is less than the nationwide average of 77; at least half of these deaths occurred in the infants' first month of life. HIV prevalence in Addis Ababa mothers was (5.2%) [7].

2.2 Study design, sample size and sampling procedures

A community based cross-sectional study was conducted from June 2016 to May 2017. Administratively, Addis Ababa is divided into 10 Sub-cities and 116 Woredas. According to 2012 CSA, there are about around 700,000 households. Three sub-cities (Gulele, Kirkos, and Lideta) and seven Woredas within these sub-cities were selected randomly. Health extension workers from each Woredas using systematic random sampling technique selected 50–70 households. The proportional allocation value, which was used for selection, was calculated by dividing the total number of households in the study area to the total number of selected households. In the end, 454 non-pregnant apparently healthy mothers were included in this study.

2.3 Data collection and laboratory investigations

Five milliliter of venous blood was collected and transported to the laboratory, where it was allowed to clot. Then, serum was separated by centrifugation at room temperature at 3000 rpm for four minutes, and then it was stored at −20°C until further use.

The principal investigator used a structured interview to collect data on socio-demographic variables and associated risk factors from the study participants. Principal investigator collected the data.

Sandwich Elisa was used to measure serum level HBsAg, Anti-HBc, and anti-HCV in all samples Bio-Rad ELISA kits were used for this study [8].

2.4 Data processing and analysis

Data entry and analysis was done using SPSS version 20.0. Chi-square test was used to determine the association between serological results and different hepatitis infection associated factors. In addition, it was used to compare categorical data, to evaluate the difference in prevalence between groups in the bivariate logistic analysis, and to determine statistical significance. To determine the association between the data obtained from the questionnaire and the laboratory results, odds ratios (ORs) and their corresponding 95% confidence intervals (CIs) were calculated using logistic regression analysis. A p-value <0.05 was considered as statistically significant.

2.5 Quality assurance

Standard operating procedures were followed during blood sample collection, processing, and analysis of data. All ELISA experiments were conducted according to the manufacturer's instruction. The performance of Monolisa™ HBsAg ULTRA was determined using test samples. A sensitivity of 100% and a specificity of

99.94% were recorded. The Monolisa™ Anti-HBc PLUS test resulted in 99.53% sensitivity and 99.5% specificity. The Monolisa™ HCV Ag-Ab ULTRA assay had 100% sensitivity and 99.83% specificity. According to the manufacturer's instruction, positive samples were tested in duplicates before final interpretation. In addition, positive and negative controls were run as the test runs.

2.6 Ethical considerations

The study received ethical approval from Ethical Review Committee and Institutional Review Board (IRB) of Addis Ababa University, College of Health Sciences, Department of Microbiology, Immunology and Parasitology and the Armauer Hansen Research Institute (AHRI). Support letter was obtained from Addis Ababa Health Bureau.

3. Results

3.1 Socio-demographic characteristics

A total of 454 mothers were involved in this study and the mean age of the study subjects was 32.75 ± 5.79 (SD) years, (range: 20 to 57 years). Majority of the mothers belonged to the 30–34 age group (33.5%), followed by 25–29 (25.1%) and 35–39 (25.1%) age group. Further, most (81.7%) of the study participants were married (**Table 1**).

3.2 Prevalence of HBV and HCV infection

Overall, 42.3% (95% CI: 39.5–46.1%) of apparently healthy mothers were positive for HBsAg, HBcAb or HCV antibody. The sero-prevalence for HBsAg was 17/454 (3.7%), while it was 165/454 (36.3%) for HBcAb and 9/454 (2.0%) for anti-HCV. 17/454 (3.7%) of the study participants were positive for both HBsAg and HBcAb. The prevalence of HBV and HCV infection segregated by age can be found in **Table 2**.

3.3 Risk factors associated with HBV and HCV infections

A positive association was observed between HBsAg seropositivity and participants' number of households ($p = 0.017$), history of liver diseases $p = 0.01$), history of jaundice ($p = 0.00$), and family history of liver disease ($p = 0.04$) at 95% confidence interval. Among participants with history of liver disease ($n = 31$), history of jaundice ($n = 9$), and family history of hepatitis ($n = 38$), the prevalence of HBsAg was 13.9%, 30.8% and 10.5% respectively. On the other hand, age, level of education, marital status, occupation, alcohol consumption habits, caring for hepatitis patients, history of operation or cesarean section, history of female genital mutilation, history of sharp injury, history of blood transfusion, history of ear-piercing, dental procedure, having multiple sexual partner, and history of abortion, did not have significant association with having hepatitis B virus infection.

In addition, binary and multivariate logistic regressions were used to determine the association between the HBV associated risk factors with HBV infection. Few predictor variables showed statistically significant association with HBV infections. Mothers with a history of hepatitis were 5.5 times more likely to be HBV positive than mothers who had no such history (AOR = 5.5; CI (1.8–16.5); $p = 0.003$).

Socio-demographic characteristics		Numbers	Percentage (%)
Age group	20–24	21	4.6
	25–29	114	25.1
	30–34	152	33.5
	35–39	114	25.1
	40–44	34	7.5
	45–49	14	3.1
	50–54	3	0.7
	55–59	2	0.4
Education	Illiterate	52	11.5
	1–8	260	57.3
	9–12	106	23.4
	≥College	36	7.9
Marital status	Married	371	81.7
	Unmarried	9	2.0
	Divorced	67	14.8
	widowed	7	1.5
Occupation	Housewife	249	54.9
	Employed	57	12.5
	Daily laborer	55	12.1
	Private	93	20.8
Family size	1–4	194	42.5
	5–6	210	46.2
	≥7	50	11.0
Total		454	100

Table 1.
Socio-demographic characteristics of study participants.

Mothers who had a history of jaundice (AOR = 17.8 CI; (4.0–75.5); p = 0.03) were 17.8 times more likely to be HBV positive than their counterparts. Statistically significant association was observed between having contact with HBV infected household members and HBV infection (P = 0.05). Mothers who had previous history of household contact were 3.2 times more likely to have infection with HBV than those without previous history of household contact (AOR = 3.2; CI (1.0–10.4); P = 0.05) (**Table 3**).

Participants' age group (p = 0.012), marital status (p = 0.05), caring for hepatitis patient (p = 0.01), blood transfusion history (p = 0.03), history of jaundice (p = 0.00), and family history of liver disease (p = 0.012) were significantly associated with HCV infection (**Table 4**). However, previous history of dental procedure, body tattooing, having multiple sexual partner, body piercing with sharp objects, and history of surgical procedure showed no significant association with having hepatitis C virus infection. In addition, HCV associated factors and their association with HCV infection was determined using binary and multivariate logistic regression. History of jaundice (AOR = 19.2; CI (3.5–104.9); p = 0.02) and alcohol consumption habit (AOR = 6.9; CI (1.3–37.0); p = 0.02) _were significantly associated with HCV positivity at 95% confidence interval. In the multivariate analysis,

Socio-demographic characteristics		Numbers	HBsAg Positive (%)	HBcAb Positive (%)	HCV Positive (%)
Age group	20–24	21	0(0.0)	6(28.6)	0(0.0)
	25–29	114	8(7.0)	34(29.9)	1(0.9)
	30–34	152	7(4.6)	55(36.2)	4(2.6)
	35–39	114	2(1.8)	40(35.1)	3(2.6)
	40–44	34	0(0.0)	19(55.9)	0(0.0)
	45–49	14	0(0.0)	8(57.1)	0(0.0)
	50–54	3	0(0.0)	2(66.7)	1(33.3)
	55–59	2	0(0.0)	1(50.0)	0(0.0)
Education	Illiterate	52	0(0.0)	11(21.2)	1(2.0)
	1–8	260	12(4.6)	97(37.3)	4(1.5)
	9–12	106	3(2.8)	43(41.0)	3(2.8)
	≥College	36	2(5.6)	14(38.9)	1(2.8)
Marital status	Married	371	16(4.3)	137(37.2)	4(1.1)
	Unmarried	9	1(11.1)	2(22.2)	0(0.0)
	Divorced	67	0(0.0)	24(35.8)	4(6.0)
	widowed	7	0(0.0)	1(28.6)	1(14.3)
Occupation	Housewife	249	11(4,5	92(36.9)	4(1.6)
	Employed	57	0(0.0)	23(40.4)	1(1.8)
	Daily laborer	55	4(7.3)	16(29.1)	2(3.6)
	Private	93	2(2.2)	34(36.6)	2(2.2)
Family size	1–4	194	3(1.5)	66(34.0)	2(1.0)
	5–6	210	9(4.3)	77(36.7)	7(3.3)
	≥7	50	5(10.0)	22(44.0)	0(0.0)
Total		454	17(3.7)	165(36.3)	9(2.0)

Table 2.
The prevalence of HBsAg, HBcAb and anti-HCV antibodies segregated by socio-demographic characteristics.

after adjustment for all other confounding variables, age group, marital status, history of blood transfusion and family history of liver disease has no impact on the acquisition of HCV infection as shown in **Table 4**.

4. Discussion

HBV and HCV infections are significant health problems around the globe. Both infections are associated with a broad range of clinical presentations ranging from clinically asymptomatic, acute hepatitis to chronic hepatitis and liver cirrhosis [9]. Population based serological studies conducted on viral hepatitis have demonstrated the diversity of epidemiological patterns with regard to the risk of acquiring infection related to personal attributes, place and risk distribution [10]. Screening asymptomatic people is important for early diagnosis and intervention, which may improve health outcomes and enhance our understanding of diseases transmission pattern [10].

S. No	Variables	HBsAg test result		COR (CI) 95%	AOR (CI) 95%	P-value
		Positive %	Negative			
1.	Diagnosis history of hepatitis Yes No	5(13.9) 12(2.9)	31 406	5.5(1.8–16) 1.0(reference)	5.4 (1.8–16.5)	0.03
2.	Caring of hepatitis patients Yes No	2(4.8) 15(3.6)	40 397	1.3(0.3–6.0) 1.0(reference)		0.72
3.	Operation Yes No	4(2.5) 13(4.4)	153 284	1.7(0.6–5.0) 1.0(reference)		0.34
4.	Sharp injury Yes No	10(4.2) 7(3.2)	227 210	1.3(0.5–3.6) 1.0(reference)		0.57
5.	Blood transfusion Yes No	2(2.7) 15(3.5)	25 412	2.3(0.5–10.6) 1.0(reference)		0.29
6.	History of jaundice Yes No	4(30.8) 13(3.0)	9 428	14.6(4.0–54) 1.0(reference)	17.8 (4–75.8)	0.03
7.	Tattoo Yes No	3(3.4) 14(3.8)	86 351	1.2(0.33–4.13) 1.0(reference)		0.82
8.	Ear-piercing Yes No	16(3.6) 1(7.7)	425 12	1.2(0.06–3.7) 1.0(reference)		0.46
9.	Dental procedure Yes No	5(3.2) 12(4.3)	152 285	1.2(0.27–2.3) 1.0(reference)		0.66
10.	Multiple sexual partner Yes No	4(5.8) 13(3.4)	65 374	1.3(0.25–7.1) 1.0(reference)		0.75
11.	Family history of hepatitis Yes No	4(9.5) 13(3.2)	38 399	3.2(1.0–10.4) 1.0(reference)	4.3 (1.5–11)	0.05
12.	History of abortion Yes No	3(2.2) 14(4.4)	136 301	2.0(0.2–3.4) 1.0(reference)		0.25
13.	Vaccine Yes No	0 17	4 433	0.0 1.0(reference)		0.99

Table 3.
Association between different risk factors and HBV infection.

The results from this study revealed 3.7% sero-prevalence of HBsAg, which lies within the established standard intermediate endemicity of hepatitis B prevalence [11]. Even though this finding in agreement with the WHO intermediate level of

	HCV test result				
Variables	**Positive (%)**	**Negative (%)**	**COR(CI)95%**	**AOR(CI) 95%**	**P value**
Marital status Married Unmarried Divorced Widowed	4(1.1) 0(0.0) 4(6.0) 1(14.3)	367(98.9) 9(100) 63(94.0) 6(85.7)	1.0 NA 5.8(1.4–23.8) 1.5(1.48–15.4)	9.3(1.5–58.8) 34.5(1.2– 100.0)	0.01 - 0.01 0.004
Caring of hepatitis patient Yes No	3(7.1) 6(1.5)	39(92.9) 406(98.5)	5.2(1.25–21.6) 1.0		0.59
Blood transfusion Yes No	2(7.7) 7(1.7)	24(92.3) 421(98.3)	5.0(1.0–25.4) 1.0		0.21
History of jaundice Yes No	2(8.3) 7(1.6)	11(91.7) 434(98.4)	11.3(2.1–60.6) 1.0	19.2(3.5– 104.9) 1.0	0.02
Family history of liver hepatitis Yes No	3(7.1) 6(1.5)	39(92.9) 406(98.5)	5.2(1.2–21.6) 1.0		0.72
Alcohol consumption Yes No	4(6.7) 5(1.3)	56(93.3) 389(98.7)	5.6(1.5–21.3) 1.0	6.9(1.3–37.0) 1.0	0.03
Total %	9(2.0)	445(98.0)			454

Table 4.
Association between risk factors and HCV infection.

endemicity, it may not represent the whole community. Because, this study mainly focuses on apparently healthy mothers in Addis Ababa, who represent only female populations; and it needs more inclusive sample from both sexes in order to argue the WHO established endemicity classifications. This result compares well with the results of a study conducted in Jimma on 493 pregnant women, where the seroprevalence was3.7% [12], and a study done in Addis Ababa on delivering women, which had sero-prevalence of 3.0% [13], and studies done in Woldia and south Gondar on diabetes and non-diabetic patients, where the seroprevalence for both was 3.7% [14]. The reported HBsAg prevalence of this study was higher than what was reported in studies conducted in Dessie on healthy female blood donors (1.5%) [15], in Addis Ababa on Public Health Centers cleaners (3.57%) [5], and in Jimma on blood donors 2.1% [16]. In contrast, it was lower than what was reported in studies conducted documented in Dessie on pregnant women (4.9%) [17], in Gondar, Bahir Dar, Dessie and Mekelle on blood donors (6.2%) [18], Shashemene (5.7%) [19], Ghana (10.6%) [20], and in Addis Ababa on the community (6.2%) [21]. The observed discrepancies in HBV distribution across different geographical locations might be attributed by variation in socio-demographic characteristics of the study population, such as socio-cultural environment, traditional practices, sexual practices, medical exposure, and the difference in hepatitis and other underlined disease epidemiology. Moreover, the variation could also be due to circulating genotypes, which is responsible for disease severity as well as treatment responses, methodological difference (test method, study design etc.), the level of awareness, and behavioral differences for the potential risk factors of HBV infection.

The overall sero-prevalence of HCV (2.0%) in this study is similar to a study conducted in Gabon (2.1%) [22], a study conducted in Sudan (1.9%) [23], sero-prevalence of the general population of Ethiopia (2.0%) [24], a study conducted in Poland (1.9%) [25] and a study conducted in northern Ethiopia volunteer testing and counseling center (2.0%) [26]. This finding was also comparable with other reports found in health center cleaners in Addis Ababa (1.59%) [5] and in blood banks at Gondar, Bahirdar, Dessie and Mekele (1.7%) [15].

In contrast, this finding was higher in a report from Dessie blood bank 0.39% [15], Jimma adult blood donors 0.2% [17], Debretabor hospital among HIV patients 1.3% [25], Arba Minch blood bank, in southern Ethiopia 0.0% [24], in Dessie among pregnant mothers was 0.8% [27], 0.19% in Indian women [28], and in Nigerian pregnant women 1.39% [29]. Moreover, our finding was lower than what was reported in studies from Gondar (5%) [30], Hawassa (6%), Kigali (5.2%), Rwanda [31], and Ghana (7.7%) [32]. These differences may be attributed to difference in sensitivity and specificity of methods used, e.g. ELISA vs. Rapid test. Another reason for these differences could be using different study designs. Usually, facility based study designs have overestimation because their population is composed of people that have already observed some of the symptoms of the infection. Sampling technique: those convenient sampling techniques usually are subjected to bias etc.), population variation, types of risk exposure and sample size that have a great effect on the result different studies.

In this study, most of socio-demographic variables were not associated with HCV infection. However, caring for hepatitis patients and history of jaundice were significantly associated with the occurrence of HCV infection. These findings were supported by a study conducted in Ethiopian public hospitals [30]. In the present study, no statistical significant differences were observed for HBV and HCV infections in terms of age, sex, occupation and educational status. This study was supported by a study reported in Amhara regional state general populations [33] and a study done in Felege Hiwot Referral Hospital, northwest Ethiopia [34].

The highest prevalence of HBsAg was detected among apparently healthy mothers, who were 25–29 or 30–34 years old. This was in agreement with studies conducted in Shashemene General Hospital, southern Ethiopia; Shenyang, China; Debretabor hospital, South Gondar, Northwest Ethiopia; Addis Ababa, Ethiopia [9, 30, 35, 36], and Nigeria [29]. The observed high prevalence of HBV positivity among younger age group could be due to h the high probability of exposure to high risk health behaviors.

The present study investigated the association of HBV infection prevalence and level of education. Higher prevalence was observed among those with primary level of education. This finding was in agreement with previous study conducted in Ethiopia among pregnant women [36]. History of liver disease, history of jaundice, and family history of liver disease were significantly associated with HBV infection and were important predictors of HBV infection. These findings were supported by a study conducted in Bahirdar [37], in Debretabor hospital [27], Gondar hospital, [29], and in Karachi, Pakistan [38].

5. Conclusion

The present study showed 3.7% and 2.0% for HBV and HCV infection prevalence, respectively. This result was an intermediate prevalence of HBV and HCV infection among apparently healthy mothers. This was in line with World Health Organization's regional HBV and HCV infection burdens [4, 9].

In our study setting, there was intermediate level of HBV and HCV prevalence apparently healthy mothers. Therefore, there is a need for timely intervention strategies to alleviate the burden of HBV and HCV infection in this community. This prevalence rate also calls for additional efforts regarding active screening and vaccination for young adults and public health education campaigns in the media to promote better awareness of viral hepatitis risk factors.

In this study, mothers within the ages of 24–29 and 30–34 had the two highest prevalence of HBV, 7.0% and 4.6% respectively. It may be at high risk and serves as a reservoir which requires routine screening and vaccine schedules (for HBV) may be important for those high risk groups.

This shows higher level of carrier status in mothers at reproductive age. This might increase risk of mother-to-infant transmission in the study areas.

Among the assessed variables and clinical presentations, previous history of liver disease, history of jaundice, and family history of liver disease were significantly associated with HBV infections. On the other hand, marital status, consumption of alcohol, and history of jaundice were significantly associated with the occurrence of HCV infection.

Scaling up of screening of pregnant and non-pregnant mothers for HBV and HCV infections and provision of health education about the risk factors, the mode of transmissions, and prevention are recommended. Population based studies with additional serological markers and molecular techniques are required to design a working strategy for evidence-based intervention. Therefore, screening apparently healthy mothers is an important tool in early diagnosis and intervention.

Acknowledgements

The Ministry of Health through the Clinical Research Capacity Building program at the Armauer Hansen Research Institute (AHRI) funded the study. I would like to acknowledge all AHRI laboratory staff for their technical and administrative support. Further, I would like to extend my thanks and appreciation to the study participants and health extension workers in Addis Ababa.

Competing interests

There was no conflict of interest between the author and other parties.

Author details

Habtamu Biazin Kebede* and Seifegebriel Teshome
Department of Microbiology, Immunology and Parasitology, Addis Ababa University, Addis Ababa, Ethiopia

*Address all correspondence to: habtamu.biazin@aau.edu.et

References

[1] World Health Organization. Prevention and control of viral hepatitis infection: framework for global action. 2012.

[2] Saeed U, Waheed Y, and Ashraf, M. Hepatitis B and hepatitis C viruses: A review of viral genomes, viral induced host immune responses, genotypic distributions and worldwide epidemiology. Asian Pacific Journal of Tropical Disease 2014, 4(2): 88-96. doi: 10.1016/S2222-1808(14)60322-4

[3] Madhava V, Burgess C, Drucker E. Epidemiology of chronic hepatitis C virus infection in sub-Saharan Africa. The Lancet infectious diseases 2005. 2(5):293-302.

[4] World Health Organization. Department of Communicable diseases surveillance and response. Hepatitis B. World Health Organization Fact Sheets 2006 (WHO/CDS/EPR/LYO/2006.2).

[5] Mekonnen A, Desta K and Damtew E. Prevalence of HBV, HCV and Associated Risk Factors among Cleaners at Selected Public Health Centers in Addis Ababa, Ethiopia. International Journal of Basic and Applied Virology 2015. 4(1): 35-40

[6] Central statistical authority, ORC Macro. Ethiopia Demographic and Health Survey, 2012. Key indicators.

[7] Central Statistical Agency of Ethiopia demographic and Health Survey. Key Indicators Report 2016.

[8] Hwang SH, Oh HB, Kim HS, and Lee EY. Evaluation of HBs Ag, HCV and HIV Ag-ab assays using bio-rad elite microplate analyzer. The Korean Journal of laboratory medicine 2006. 26(6): 436-441.

[9] World Health Organization. Guidelines for the screening, care and treatment of persons with chronic hepatitis B and C infection 2017.World Health Organization fact sheet.

[10] Wolfgang T, Jeffrey A, and Karen E. Hepatitis C virus quantification: Optimization of strategies for detecting low-level viremia. Journal of Clinical Microbiology 2000; 38(2):888-891.

[11] Simmonds P. Variability of hepatitis C virus. Hepatology 2006. 21(2): 570-583.

[12] Awole M, Gebre-Selassie S. Seroprevalence of HBsAg and its risk factors among pregnant women in Jimma, Southwest Ethiopia. Ethiopian Journal Health Development 2005.19(1):45-50.

[13] Tegegne D, Desta K, Tegbaru B, and Tilahun T. Seroprevalence and transmission of hepatitis B virus among delivering women and their new born in selected health facilities, Addis Ababa, Ethiopia: A cross sectional study. BioMedicine Central Research Notes 2014.7:239.

[14] Mekonnen D, Gebre-Selassie S, Fantaw S, Hunegnaw A, and Mihret A. Prevalence of hepatitis B virus in patients with diabetes mellitus: A comparative cross sectional study at Woldiya general hospital, Ethiopia. Pan African Medical Journal 2014. 17(1).78-81

[15] Sharew B, Mulu A, Teka B, and Tesfaye T. Frequency of hepatitis B and C virus infections among blood donors in Northeast Ethiopia. Current Research Microbiology Biotechnology 2015. 3(2): 614-617.

[16] Yami A, Alemseged F, Hassen A. Hepatitis B and C viruses' infections and their association with human immunodeficiency virus: A cross-sectional study among blood donors in

Ethiopia. Ethiopian journal of health sciences 2011. 21(1):67-75.

[17] .Seid M, Gelaw B, Assefa A. Sero-prevalence of HBV and HCV infections among pregnant women attending antenatal care clinic at Dessie Referral Hospital, Ethiopia. Advance Life Sciences Health 2014. 1(2):109-120.

[18] Gelaw B and Mengitsu Y. The prevalence of HBV, HCV and malaria parasites among blood donor in Amhara and Tigray regional states. Ethiopian Journal of Health Development 2008. 22(1):3-7.

[19] Negero A, Sisay Z, Medhin G. Prevalence of hepatitis B surface antigen (HBsAg) among visitors of Shashemene general hospital voluntary counseling and testing center. BioMedicine Central Research Notes 2011. 4:35.

[20] Cho Y, Bonsu G, Akoto-Ampaw A, et al. The prevalence and risk factors for hepatitis B surface Ag positivity in pregnant women in eastern region of Ghana. Gut and liver 2012. 6(2): 235.

[21] Abebe A, Nokes DJ, Dejene A, Enquselassie F, Messele T, and Cutts FT. Seroepidemiology of hepatitis B virus in Addis Ababa, Ethiopia: Transmission patterns and vaccine control. Epidemiology and infection 2013. 131(01):757-770.

[22] Ndong-Atome GR, Makuwa M, Njouom R, et al. Hepatitis C virus prevalence and genetic diversity among pregnant women in Gabon, Central Africa. Bio Medicine Central infectious diseases 2008. 8(1):82.

[23] Indris KH and Elamin BK. Seroprevalence of hepatitis B (HBsAg) and hepatitis C (anti-HCV) viruses among Sudanese patients with HIV/TB Co-infection. International Journal of Information Research and Review 2015. 2(06):765-768.

[24] Frommel D, Tekle-Haimanot R, Berhe N, Aussel L, Verdier M, Preux PM, Denis F. A survey of antibodies to hepatitis C virus in Ethiopia. The American journal of tropical medicine and hygiene 1993. 49(4):435-439.

[25] Flisiak R, Halota W, Horban A, Juszczyk J, Pawlowska M, and Simon K. Prevalence and risk factors of HCV infection in Poland. European Journal of gastroenterology & hepatology 2011. 23(12), 1213-1217.

[26] Atsbaha AH, Dejen TA, Belodu R, Getachew K, Saravanan M, Wasihun AG. Seroprevalence and associated risk factors for hepatitis C virus infection among voluntary counseling testing and anti-retroviral treatment clinic attendants in Adwa hospital, northern Ethiopia. BioMedicine Central research notes 2016. 9(1):121.

[27] Wondimeneh Y, Alem M, Asfaw F, Belyhun Y. HBV and HCV seroprevalence and their correlation with CD4 cells and liver enzymes among HIV positive individuals at University of Gondar Teaching Hospital, Northwest Ethiopia. Virology Journal 2013. 10(1):171.

[28] Mehta KD, Antala S, Mistry M, Goswami Y. Seropositivity of hepatitis B, hepatitis C, syphilis, and HIV in antenatal women in India. The Journal of Infection in Developing Countries 2013. 7(11):832-837.

[29] Esan AJ, Omisakin CT, Ojo-Bola T, Owoseni MF, Fasakin KA, Ogunleye AA. Sero-prevalence of hepatitis B and hepatitis C virus co-infection among pregnant women in Nigeria. American Journal of Biomedical Research 2014. 2(1):11-15

[30] Balew M, Moges F, Yismaw G, Unakal C. Assessment of hepatitis B and C virus infections and associated risk

factors in HIV infected patients at Debretabor hospital, South Gondar, Northwest Ethiopia. Asian Pacific Journal of Tropical Disease 2014.4(1):1-7.

[31] Rusine J, Ondoa P, Asiimwe-Kateera B, et al. High seroprevalence of HBV and HCV infection in HIV-infected adults in Kigali, Rwanda. PloS one 2013. 8(5):e63303.

[32] Ephraim R, Donko I, Sakyi SA, Ampong J, Agbodjakey H. Seroprevalence and risk factors of hepatitis B and hepatitis C infections among pregnant women in the Asante Akim north municipality of the Ashanti region, Ghana; a cross sectional study. African Health Sciences 2015. 15(3):709-713.

[33] Abera B, Adem Y, Yimer M, Mulu W, Zenebe Y, Mekonnen Z. Community seroprevalence of hepatitis B, C and human immunodeficiency virus in adult population in Gojjam zones, Northwest Ethiopia. Virology journal 2017. 14(1):21.

[34] Molla S, Munshea A, and Nibret E. Seroprevalence of hepatitis B surface antigen and anti HCV antibody and its associated risk factors among pregnant women attending maternity ward of FelegeHiwot referral hospital, Northwest Ethiopia: A cross-sectional study. Virology Journal 2015.12:204.

[35] Ding Y, Sheng Q, Ma L, Dou X. Chronic HBV infection among pregnant women and their infants in Shenyang, China. Virology journal 2013. 10(1):17.

[36] Desalegn Z, Wassie L, Beyene HB, Mihret A, Ebstie YA. Hepatitis B and human immunodeficiency virus co-infection among pregnant women in resource-limited high endemic setting, Addis Ababa, Ethiopia: Implications for prevention and control measures. European journal of medical research 2016. 21(1):16.

[37] Zenebe Y, Mulu W, Yimer M, Abera B. Sero-prevalence and risk factors of hepatitis B virus and human immunodeficiency virus infection among pregnant women in Bahir Dar city, Northwest Ethiopia: A cross sectional study. BioMedicine Central infectious diseases 2014. 14(1):118.

[38] Jafri W, Jafri N, Yakoob J, Islam M, Tirmizi S, Jafar T, Akhtar S, Hamid S, Shah H,. and Nizami, S.. hepatitis B and C: Prevalence and risk factors associated with seropositivity among children in Karachi, Pakistan. BMC Infectious Diseases 2006.6(1):101.